RESHAPE YOUR BODY

USING CALORIE CYCLING DIET AND SPECIAL EXERCISES

By Roman Malkov, M.D.

ISBN: 978-0-615-18123-3

This book is not intended to replace the services of a physician or dietician. Any application of the recommendations set forth in the following pages is at the reader's discretion. The reader should consult with his or her own physician or dietician concerning the recommendations in this book.

Preface

In my practice as a sports medicine nutritionist, I see many people over the age of 35 who exercise regularly and watch their diet. They try commercial diet products, personal trainers or nutritionists, and nothing happens. They wonder why they cannot achieve the lean body they seek. I also have patients who think they can look as athletic as the models in the commercials simply by changing their diet.

Many of my patients have been taking fat burners, exercising religiously and dieting by skipping meals, all at once, and still have a hard time trying to get in shape. That is not because they are lazy or did not try; it is simply because no one ever told them what to do and how to do it right. What they did not realize is that long-term calorie restriction was making the situation worse.

I always try to explain to these patients that their metabolism is working against them. As we age, merely dieting does not give us the results we want because our bodies go through hormonal changes that slows the metabolism. That makes it hard to achieve goals such as fat loss or muscle building. What works for an 18 year old does not necessarily would work when you are 38-years old. We can no longer achieve the look we want without addressing these metabolic changes.

Look at it this way. One day about the time you celebrated your 35th birthday anniversary, you started to notice something about yourself. You no longer had the strength of a speeding locomotive. You could

3

no longer leap tall buildings at a single bound. In fact, you could no longer see through a brick wall. Worst of all, you've been on a diet and nothing is working. Your body resists all efforts at weight loss, no matter how hard you try. Your goal of achieving or maintaining that athletic look suddenly becomes remote. How do you overcome these and other obstacles in getting back that beautiful body? At this point, The Calorie Cycling Diet becomes the main tool to restore your body and strengthen your soul.

In this book, I attempt to address the problem of the slowdown in metabolism that comes naturally with age. I show how using a proven, scientific approach will increase metabolism and improve overall health. This approach was developed as a result of many years of nutritional experiments with professional athletes in Russia. I have modified this technique to suit the needs of ordinary people. The result is that the most powerful diet was born. The Calorie Cycling Diet — as none of the other diets — can make you look and feel athletic, a few years younger and provoke jealous looks from your best friends.

Let me start with this statement:

We eat more than our bodies need because we have established unhealthy and gluttonous eating habits.

3 Simple Concepts

There are three basic concepts;

1. You must alternate between normal calories (normal-cal) days and low calories (low-cal) days. That's main principle of the Calorie Cycling Diet.

2. On **normal calories days**, you should perform strength training. This is done by lifting weights using dumbbells or with resistance training machines set at heavy weight. Focus on muscles in the areas where you want them to be bigger, for example shoulders.

3. On **low-cal days**, you must perform aerobic exercises. Make sure that you exercise muscles in the areas where you want less fat, for example Manhattan Rush exercise.

Later, these concepts will be fully examined.

Say Hello to the Calorie Cycling Diet

The Proven Power of CCD

The full power of CCD — and the benefits of fat loss it provides — develops only gradually, over a period of time. The full benefits cannot show up until your insulin level comes down. That takes time to happen and it varies with each person. Some people may spend weeks before noticing the first sign of diminished insulin secretion, i.e. a diminished appetite. After that happens, your protein-rich, low-cal days will become efficient fat-loss days.

Here is what will be happening. Many years of undisciplined eating compelled your pancreas to secrete large amounts of insulin, even between meals. Freely eaten snacks, bread and sweets created a constant need for insulin secretions. How does that affect your health? Slowly but surely that kind of activity begins to wear out your pancreas, predisposing you to develop Type 2 diabetes. Along with undisciplined eating comes an array of cardiovascular complications in the heart and lungs that you begin to notice after your 40th birthday anniversary.

Why, you may ask, don't young people suffer dire consequences from gorging on carbs? The main reason is because young people generate high levels of protective hormones – human growth, thyroid and sex hormones. Second, they engage in a high level of physical activities. Because of their vigorous exercise, the sugar-water glucose in their blood burns up before it gets deposited as fat. When you are young, those surging hormones are your protective shield. When age tightens the hormone supply, the level of protection drops. That's why middle-age opens the door to disease and the age-related loss of muscle and bone.

So what are the benefits of CCD?

First, the diet reduces carbohydrate consumption. That alone gives your pancreas the luxury of a well-needed rest.

Second, after sessions of intensive exercise on normal-cal days, CCD boosts the level of anabolic hormones — HGH, thyroid hormones and testosterone. That's exactly what you need. That provides an anti-aging action. When this regimen is followed faithfully, CCD provides powerful anti-aging and health protection benefits.

Many people continue to ask me why I concentrate on carbohydrates? Why not on fat? Why not on protein?

First, carbohydrates trigger an insulin secretion, which plays an important role in building fat deposits and controlling blood sugar that influences the onset of hunger. At first, eating refined carbohydrates makes you feel full and brings on a sense of satiety. Soon after that, a new wave of hunger strikes.

Second, carbohydrates are the basis for many of our pleasure foods. We usually eat pleasure foods in such large quantities that the number of calories we consume exceeds the amount we burn for energy. Most of our pleasure foods — white bread, pasta, cookies, cakes and ice cream — contain refined carbohydrates, which quickly break down into glucose, a blood sugar and a very powerful energy source. Like nuclear fuel, refined carbohydrates — if managed properly — provide useful energy. Yet, if either is left uncontrolled, it can lead to disaster.

Bet you hadn't thought about this. When we consume refined carbohydrates, we touch off a storm reaction in our bodies. The storm sends waves of insulin coursing through the bloodstream. It takes time before insulin stabilizes and returns to its original level. During that wild time many things happen: nutrients move through cell membranes, the blood glucose level changes, resulting in a craving for more sweets. While refined carbohydrates initially give us a sense of well-being, in the long run they damage the internal organs. For example, too much insulin can result in fatty deposits on the walls of the blood vessels and that can eventually clog them and lead to hypertension, stroke, or a heart attack (myocardial infarction). We may not suffer a heart attack within seconds of eating a piece of birthday cake, but years of bingeing on refined carbohydrates can accumulate a powerful lot of damage.

Is sugar a poison? Many medical and nutritional authorities label sugar as a silent killer. Slowly but surely, sugar does kill people. When you were a child, your mother warned you about putting too much sugar on your cereal. Or drinking too much soda pop. "Sugar will make you fat," she scolded. "It'll rot your teeth. Addle your brain."

Well big surprise. No matter what you eat — be it T-bone steak, pizza, or grapefruit — all that food gets churned up there in your gut. It's called digestion. We'll learn a lot about digestion in this book. And the very first thing to know about digestion is that the busy churn down in your gut produces mainly three things — regardless of whether it came from meat, butterfat or cupcakes. These three things are fatty acids (from fat), amino acids (from protein) and glucose (from carbohydrates). Glucose is sugar water, pure and simple. In the hospital, when the nurse sticks a needle in your arm, she is preparing to feed you glucose. With a few exceptions (amino acids, vitamins, etc.) that we'll learn about in this book, that baked potato ends up as glucose in your gut. And those carbohydrates — be they angel food or devils food cake — enter your bloodstream as glucose. Obviously, something funny is going on here. So stick around for a real education in what turns our daily food into bone and muscle, ligaments and fat, blood and brains. It is important to keep in mind that a molecule of fat contains more than twice as many calories (9) as protein and carbohydrate (both 4). That's why you have to keep a gimlet eye on fat in your diet.

Here's a thing or two you should know about carbohydrates or carbs as people call them today. Highly refined carbs like pasta, sugar, bread and cake, digest almost instantly. When they hit the bloodstream, they trigger the pancreas gland to squirt a shot of insulin into the bloodstream. The purpose of the insulin is to carry that cake-turned-sugar-water to the body's cells to be used as energy or to be stored as fat. Consider insulin as a submarine carrying sugar water through a river of blood.

Our food profile consists of protein, fat, and carbohydrates. Proteins are made up of chains of amino acids, which serve as essential building blocks for muscles. Our body needs amino acids on a daily basis to rejuvenate itself. That's why amino acids are considered essential. Protein does not trigger the same insulin surge that carbs do (Picture 1). Carbs are simple sugars called saccharids, When dealing with carbs, it is important to know that there are no "essential" saccharids. In other words, your body does not need carbs for everyday survival. If you ate no carbs, you would not be deprived of any valuable nutrient, vitamin or mineral. While we can go without carbs and not get a disease, the failure to eat protein would lead to megaloblastic anemia (vitamin B-12 deficiency) and kwashiorkor, a form of malnutrition. Not eating enough fat would lead to hormonal imbalances.

9

Compare a 2,000-calorie-a-day diet based on carbohydrates with a 2,000-calorie-a-day diet based on protein. After eating a carbohydrate-rich meal, some fat deposition will take place during insulin spikes. On a protein-based diet, no insulin spike occurs and fat deposition may not take place. That is why you need to pay attention to carbohydrates in your food.

You have heard many times that if your calorie intake exceeds your calorie expenditure, the unused calories will turn to fat. In other words, if you deduct the number of calories you burn from the number of calories you eat, you have the number of calories that will turn to fat. That's not quite right. That formula fails to take into account two important storage cells — the muscle and liver glycogen depots — that can absorb a lot of calories. The Calorie Cycling Diet will teach you how to use these two "dietary storage cells" for your personal benefit. And that makes all the difference between the CCD diet and all the others.

If someone were to overeat by 200 calories a day — many of us do so routinely — by the end of the year, he or she would gain 21 pounds. In ten years, that would add up to an additional 210 pounds. If that happened, a 30-year-old man who weighed 150 pounds would exceed 800 pounds by the time he began collecting Social Security. That simply doesn't happen.

Many of my patients complain that they eat 500 to 700 fewer calories than their daily needs and lose no weight. The common practice among nutritionists is to advise the dieter to lower the calorie intake by 500 calories and expect to see a one pound fat loss each week. (A pound of fat contains 3,500 calories.) It just doesn't work that way. The body quickly lowers its Basal Metabolic Rate so the calorie-deficit disappears. As you can see, the simple mathematical calculation of input and output that we have been taught to rely on is not accurate. Our body has complex regulatory and adaptation mechanisms. The secret of the CCD diet is to work with these mechanisms — and not against them. That is what makes Calorie Cycling perform seeming miracles. Nutrition is not a precise science based on mathematics, even though many nutrition advisers would have you think so. There are mechanisms that usually are not accounted for by the conventional dieting approach. The Calorie Cycling Diet book will concentrate on one of those mechanisms — how your body handles glucose and glycogen and how you can use this knowledge to keep calories from being deposited as fat.

The Calorie Cycling Diet aims at preventing the adaptation changes that occur when someone's behavior becomes repetitious. For example, when someone consumes a calorie-restricted diet day after day for months on end, the body adjusts to a starvation-diet by lowering its metabolism. When someone performs the same exercise day after day, the body adjusts and starts hoarding calories. Knowing this allows you to take preventive action. In the book, I discuss the use of:

• Exercise to deplete muscle glycogen content and boost anabolic hormone secretion

• Supplements to increase energy and endurance, and

• Amino acids and herbs to activate the thyroid gland

These, if used in combination, are key factors in combating the negative physiological changes that accompany human aging. You might say they provide a key to the Fountain of Youth.

The Calorie Cycling Diet is most effective when coupled with regular exercise. It helps to achieve and keep a desired body shape.

- Even if you cannot find time for exercise, you still can apply the Calorie Cycling strategy to keep your body healthy.

The goal of CCD is not just to lose a few pounds of fat. Who wants to look old and skinny, like a wicked old witch? The goal CCD pursues is to lose fat by increasing the hormonal levels so you can look lean with a youthful athletic appearance, with elastic and vibrant skin, feeling energetic and capable of doing physical things that your peers are simply unable to do.

Words of Wisdom for Dieters

The instructions given here apply generally to mature men or women between the ages of 35 and 45: the most dangerous years for weight gain — be wary of weight gain during these critical years. To avoid damage resulting from severe calorie restriction, you should take action now while you still have a chance. Otherwise, it might become too late.

The readers of this book will no doubt range from vigorous adolescents in the peak of good health to senior citizens who are in want of true happiness during their golden years because of infirmity, atrophied muscles, obesity or bone loss.

Before undertaking any diet and exercise, it's wise to see your doctor first. If you are pregnant or have a history of heart problems, have had broken bones, a slipped disc or some other problem, your family physician can best give you advice based on your medical history. Then chart out a timetable of where you are now, where you would like to be in six months and your goal for the next year.

The basic 1-1 regimen is intended for novices to dieting. It works well when combined with exercise. See examples in Part II.

 To stimulate fat loss, increase your physical activity or temporarily switch to Level B and a greater number of low-cal days. That's the way to regulate your weight, enjoy good health and still have an occasional ice cream cone.

Part 1

Your Guide To Diet

4 vexing problems with calorie-restricted diets

- How do you keep your metabolism up and running?

- How do you alternate anabolism with catabolism?

- How do you eat refined carbohydrates and not become fat?

- How do you diet without exercise?

Chapter 1

Anabolism vs. Catabolism

The Problem With Calorie-Restricted Diets

A new millennium has arrived and everyone thinks they know how to diet. After all, this generation the smartest, best educated age group in the history of the world. And there are literally hundreds of diet products on the market. Yet, more than half of all Americans are overweight — many are obese. Why? Something is drastically wrong.

Remember those wonderful adolescent years when you could gulp snack foods and not worry about putting on weight? Your metabolism was active because of high hormonal levels — surplus calories were simply burned away. As you reached maturity, something called human growth hormone and thyroid hormone levels began to decline. Your metabolism rate slowed down. If daily carbohydrate intake remained at the same level, those extra calories were no longer burned as efficiently. Instead they began being stored as fat. As we age we tend to deposit more and more fat and lose more and more muscle and bone mass. And that's not good for you or anybody else. CCD is designed to stop this dual process of deterioration.

As You Age, Your Eating Habits Must Change

Can we reverse life's inevitable metabolic slowdown? Can we at least halt this aging tendency? We cannot delay the aging process dramatically, but as this book will demonstrate, we can take a few measures that help us to stay younger longer. Don't laugh: it's the only Fountain of Youth you will ever chance upon.

All fad diets have a similar idea: to reduce the number of calories the dieter consumes. What effect does that have down the road? It may not be noticeable until you spend a year on the diet. There are ample studies to show that 25 percent of dietary weight loss comes from the loss of muscle tissues. In short, losing fat is accompanied by losing muscle. Do we lose protein selectively from the muscles? The answer is a definite no. Besides muscle protein, there is a loss of connective tissue protein — those called elastin and collagen. The connective-tissue proteins are what make your skin elastic and firm. They are nature's own Botox. The loss of these tissues makes your skin sag and that creates wrinkles. The connective tissue proteins are part of joint cartilage and ligaments. The loss of it leads to developing joint pains and osteoarthrosis.

Take a look at anyone who has been on a calorie-restricted diet for a year or more. Even though they lost weight, the skin on their face is wrinkled. It is no longer elastic. In contrast, someone who is overweight boasts skin that looks healthy plump and firm. One study revealed that men who live on a calorie-restricted diet have 35 percent less testosterone compared to men who eat normally. What does that mean for those men? It means feeling tired at the end of the day, less energy and vigor, less interest in sex, fewer muscles to flex. Testosterone is one of the anabolic hormones. As we age we tend to secrete fewer and fewer anabolic hormones, losing more and more protein and bone mass. Do calorie-restricted diets help us feel and look younger? Not really. In contrast, The Calorie Cycling Diet prevents diet-related slowdown of metabolism. As you can see, if combined with a proper exercise program, CCD provides a significant anti-aging benefit.

Here's a looming problem for someone on a calorie restricted diet for prolonged period of time. They suffer from undernutrition (a form of malnutrition) and a weakening of the immune system — the body's first line of defense against cancer and infections[76]. The average American is not consuming anywhere near the amount of fruit and vegetables recommended by the American Dietary Association, even those who are not on a calorie restricted diet. What happens when the amount of food he or she eats is artificially restricted? The body does not receive adequate amounts of active nutrients, vitamins, minerals. Although no studies have been done on the influence of calorie-restricted diets on cancer rates, I would not be surprised if such a study would reveal an increased chance of getting cancer among those who live on a calorie-restricted diet for a long time.

Some may say a daily multivitamin formula will cover up for nutritional gaps. It does not. The best multivitamin and minerals formula have only a small percentage of the wide spectrum of nutrients found in natural foods, sometimes even in unnatural, chemically synthesized form. The importance of consuming a variety of foods is obvious to any nutritionist or medical doctor.

Definitions for This Chapter

To help you understand what follows, here are simple definitions for some complex nutritional terms.

Glucose (blood sugar): Glucose is a single sugar molecule (monosaccharide) related to table sugar (sucrose). Your body has a regulatory mechanism to keep its blood glucose concentration constant. When the blood glucose concentration rises, the pancreas secretes a hormone called insulin that decreases the sugar concentration by pushing the glucose into body cells. What would happen if blood glucose were not regulated? The blood concentration might reach levels at which the osmotic ingredient in glucose would attract water to the blood vessels leaving cell tissues dehydrated. That action would lead to death. On the other hand, a feeble level of blood glucose is not compatible with life because glucose must be present in blood for energy production.

Refined carbohydrates: Refined carbohydrates are the starches left when whole grains — wheat, rye, and oats — are highly refined. The process removes most of the fiber and nutrients. Wild rice is an example of a whole grain. White rice is an example of a refined carbohydrate. Carbohydrates without fiber — white bread, for instance — quickly convert into glucose which is absorbed into the blood stream causing insulin levels to skyrocket.

Because many vital nutrients are lost in processing, government regulations require that refined carbohydrates be "fortified" with vitamins and other nutrients.

Crude carbohydrates: Whole grains are cracked or cut. In other words, they are only minimally refined — they retain their fiber. That fiber slows digestion so the glucose is absorbed slowly, with less insulin secretion than is produced by the digestion of refined carbohydrates. Until modern milling was introduced in the 1880s,

18

cut grains were just about the sole source of cereals in our diet. Until the end of the 19th century, our ancestors did not have the constantly elevated levels of insulin in their blood. Neither did they suffer from arterial plaque (atherosclerosis), heart attack (myocardial infarction), stroke and diabetes, which are so prevalent today.

With the arrival of commercial food processing, our bodies also had to deal with another source of glucose, the sugar added to foods made from refined carbohydrates. After three million years of evolution, our bodies had adjusted to fructose, the type of sugar found naturally in fruits and honey. The important characteristic of fructose is that it does not trigger insulin secretion as much as other sugars do. For this reason our ancestors did not have constantly elevated levels of insulin in their blood. The ability of fructose to enter cells without the assistance of insulin today creates another problem: when consumed in large quantities — as in soft drinks — any part of fructose not used for energy converts to glucose and is deposited as fat.

We put our pancreas under extreme stress when it continually tries to secrete large amounts of insulin. When we constantly eat refined carbohydrates, our blood sugar concentration and insulin levels never drop. At some point, the pancreas is unable to handle the load. People who are genetically predisposed then begin to develop Type 2 diabetes. In the last century, the growth of this disease rose drastically and, unfortunately, it shows a tendency to continue to grow.

Metabolism — (me-TAB-o-lism) Metabolism is the sum of all chemical processes involved in life, the process by which energy is produced[57]. In living organisms, both chemical and physical processes go on continuously. There are two branches to metabolism: catabolism and anabolism. These subcategories of metabolism describe the processes that balance between each other on a daily basis. The body constantly is in the process of disintegrating and rejuvenating its tissues. The balance between catabolism and anabolism is controlled by level of Human Growth Hormone, thyroid hormone, DHEA and sex hormones.

Catabolism (ka-TAB-o-lism) Catabolism is the process by which complex structures are broken down into simple ones: glucose, amino acids and fatty acids. Catabolism is the process by which body fat is converted into the energy our bodies can use.

Consider this simple equation.

- Calories You Eat - Calories You Burn =

    Calorie Balance

When you consume fewer calories than you use, the balance becomes negative and you are in a catabolic state, a condition where catabolism dominates over anabolism. Catabolism leads to fat loss.

Anabolism (a-NAB-o-lism), the opposite of catabolism, is a constructive process. It is the process by which simple food substances — glucose, fatty acids and amino acids — are changed into living tissue: flexing biceps and fulsome lips. When you eat more calories than you burn, the balance become positive. That condition lets your body deposit fat and rejuvenate proteins, which builds muscles and connective tissue.

Let's look at how these two subcategories work together.

Picture 2. The Balance between anabolism and catabolism

Anabolism

Building of protein, fat

Energy Consumption

Catabolism

Breakdown of fat, protein

Energy Release

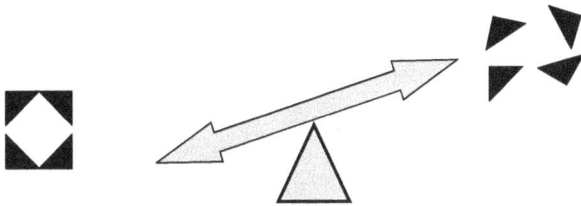

Rule 1: Losing Fat = Catabolism

- You cannot lose fat unless you are in a Negative Calorie Balance

Rule 2: Building Protein = Anabolism

- You cannot build protein (muscle and connective tissues) unless you are in a Positive Calorie Balance

Rule 3: Fat and Muscle

- You cannot lose fat and build muscle on the same day

How to Lose Fat and Build Protein

While you cannot lose fat and build protein on the same day, you can achieve both goals by alternating the days when you lose fat with the days when you build protein.

Remember

- You must alternate periods of catabolism,
  when you lose fat,
  with periods of anabolism, when your body
  builds proteins and rejuvenates its tissues.

This alternating process is the very core of The Calorie Cycling Diet. By following an eating plan that restricts calories on one day and allows consuming more calories on another day, you will not only lose fat, but you will also maintain your muscle mass and vigor by keeping your anabolism running high.

Did You Know?

- As we age, catabolism gradually overtakes anabolism

- As we age the tissue's sensitivity to insulin changes. The organs become less responsive to insulin and body adjusts by increasing insulin secretion. More insulin in the blood leads to bigger accumulation of fat.

As we age, we lose bone and muscle mass and accumulate more fat. In other words, we become flabby and obese. If we try to counteract

23

this fat gain by following a traditional diet that simply reduces calorie intake, it makes a bad situation worse. Traditional dieting slows down a metabolism that is already impaired by aging. Calorie restriction brought on by dieting slows the important rejuvenation processes taking place every day. It also accelerates the negative effects of aging: muscle loss, bone loss, wrinkle formation, and a decrease in the production of the vital anabolic hormones: Human Growth Hormone, thyroid hormone, testosterone and DHEA.

Inadequate nutrition, the reduced food-intake of diets and a sedentary, couch-potato lifestyle accelerates the impairments brought on by old age. The desirable and beneficial metabolic condition is anabolism predominance, which can be reached only with a Positive Calorie Balance — and by increasing the level of anabolic hormones. As you age, you need to speed up your metabolism so you lose fat. The Calorie Cycling Diet is the only diet that does that.

Conventional dieting leads to muscle and bone loss. It also leads to a sagged, wrinkled skin.

Important

- As we age, the approach to fat loss should be to accelerate metabolism — not to slow it as the fad diets do

❖ ❖ ❖

The Chemistry of Fat Accumulation

When someone loses weight on a calorie-restrained diet, his metabolic processes slow down — his body is trying to preserve life. Like a car running on low octane gas, the body cannot run at its best while on a calorie-restricted diet. Without adequate calories, the body produces fewer anabolic hormones — testosterone and Human Growth Hormone — which it needs to sustain youth and energy.

Consider a popular high-protein, low carbohydrate diet such as Atkins. A high-protein diet works much the same as a conventional calorie-restricted diet because you consume fewer calories than you would normally. It is difficult to consume more than 2,000 calories a day when you are eating mostly protein food. When carb-intake is restricted for an extended period, catabolism predominance leads to conditions, such as joint problems, depletion of calcium and loss of proteins. After a few months on these diets, people detect these problems themselves and become concerned. How healthy is that?

Here are just a few of the negative consequences that result from long-term calorie restriction:

- Slow metabolism — the opposite of the desired goal

- Lack of libido — fewer sex hormones are produced

- Depression – low testosterone

- Wrinkles and sagged skin— loss of connective tissue proteins

- Joint pain — the breakdown of cartilage and slow repair

- Muscle loss

- Accelerated osteoporosis – slow bone repair

A few words about osteoporosis. Some of my patients, age 50 or more, who are trying to lose fat ask me if it is healthy to go on the Atkins or South Beach diet. Here is what I tell them. Osteoporosis is often called the silent disease. For years, you can lose bone density without realizing what's happening. The first sign might be when you step down a stairway and your hip gives way, shattering a bone weakened by the silent loss of calcium.

Evidence of a possible link between low-carb diets such as the Atkins Diet and bone loss was published in the *American Journal of Kidney Diseases*. Researchers doing a six-week trial found two things: participants' loss of calcium in urine increased during the study and their bodies did not compensate for it by increasing the absorption of calcium from other sources. Subjects' calcium balance dropped by as much as 130 milligrams daily. By comparison, a glass of low-fat cow's milk contains around 225 milligrams of calcium.

If continued over a number of years, the loss of calcium could increase the risk of osteoporosis. "People may lose weight on this diet, but this study shows that this is not a healthy way to lose weight," said Dr. Chia-ying Wang, a co-author of the study.

This is a good time for a lesson about calcium and osteoporosis There is more calcium in your body than any other mineral. About 99 percent of this calcium is locked up in your bones and teeth, which is what makes them strong. The remaining fraction is distributed throughout the body, and this calcium is essential to the proper functioning of every cell in your body. Calcium is vital to all life processes. The heartbeat, muscle contractions, the hormone system, the functioning of your brain, your eyes and ears — all depend on calcium. It plays a critical role in blood clotting and cell division.

Calcium requires magnesium to make tooth enamel and it needs phosphorous to make bones. Our bones are about 40 percent calcium and 45 percent phosphorus. Vitamin D is needed for the absorption and use of calcium. A deficiency of Vitamin D reduces the calcium available to your body. The need for vitamins and minerals is inter-related.

There is calcium in the intercellular fluid that surrounds body cells. Inside of each cell, the calcium level is only one ten-thousandth of the level outside the cell. When a tiny amount of calcium enters a cell, it becomes a powerful signal to control cell activities: metabolism, growth, contraction. Without that calcium your body would shut down. Calcium achieves its wide spectrum of activities by using a see-saw control mechanism — with a hormone made from Vitamin D,

Calcium Bank: Make Your Deposit by Age 25

The greatest need for calcium is during the young and growing years. Special attention should be given to calcium intake until age 25. So critical is the calcium balance that the human body does not depend on your eating habits to offset calcium fluctuations owing to normal wear and tear. Instead, a calcium thermostat — the parathyroid gland — secretes hormones to regulate the concentration of calcium in the blood and intercellular fluids. If there is not enough calcium, the thermostat orders a withdrawal from the bone bank. That's drastic.

It is well to build up the equity in your calcium bank early in life. By age 35, you will start losing more bone than you make (even though people rejuvenate bone tissue daily). If you don't attain peak bone mass by age 25, the downhill slide will be even faster. The alarming fact for Americans is that their calcium intake is often below the US RDA. A low-calorie, low-exercise diet — for example, Atkins without exercise — forces the body to excrete calcium.

Dairy products are unpopular among today's adolescents. Large numbers of young girls are obsessed with watching their caloric intake. At the same time, the beverage industry promotes milk as babyish and soda pop as being cool. The youngsters drink colored fizz-water fortified with naked calories but no nutrients. As a result, fewer than one in six adolescent girls get half the US RDA of 1,200 mg a day of calcium.

Osteoporosis is an incurable but treatable bone disease that affects half of American women over the age of 45. Gulping calcium tablets cannot cure osteoporosis. Nothing can. The key is prevention, which includes adequate calcium intake early in life and plenty of exercise throughout life. The best sources of calcium are milk, cheese, dairy products, dark green leafy vegetables, dried beans and peas. Also lime-processed corn tortillas, the soft bones of canned fish and the tips of poultry leg bones. Put these foods on your approved list.

What other preventive measures can you take?

• The first one is calcium supplements.

• The second one is exercise.

Numerous studies show that repetitive and regular load on bones (especially jumping) makes the bones stronger, increases calcium turnover and promotes overall bone strength. (If you are not in peak physical condition, get into jumping exercises slowly, over a period of weeks or months. You may wish to start by jumping rope for a few minutes a day.)

Using diet pills and skin patches to suppress appetite is a popular way to lose fat employed by the credulous — people who would believe anything. Pills and patches don't work in the long term. As soon as people stop taking them, their appetite returns along with the lost fat. So what is a solution? Living on diet pills for the rest of your life?

- If you want to lose fat in a healthy way,

  you should alternate between catabolism

  and anabolism.

How do you make anabolism dominate over catabolism? Exercise with heavy weights and eat enough calories to force your body release anabolic hormones.

Catabolism allows you to lose weight by reducing your calorie intake. The extra energy produced by anabolism synthesizes hormones and other complex substances and gives your body a youth-preserving boost. During anabolism, your body can repair broken chains of proteins more effectively. It can renew proteins, such as those in the skin. Without these extra calories, the rate of repair of elastin and collagen slows and the skin loses its firmness and elasticity. If we don't take measures to counteract this process, we begin to look old and thin. The Calorie Cycling Diet allows you to achieve a healthy balance between trimming off fat and keeping that gleaming young body longer.

❖ ❖ ❖

The Role of Hormones

Biochemists understand the process of glucose metabolism, but they aren't clear on why some people can bolt down large amounts of sugar and refined carbohydrates and not gain weight. Why, for instance, can a 16-year-old swill pizza, ice cream and cookies, and gulp 32-ounce cola drinks — consuming more than 3,000 calories a day — and still maintain a lithe five-percent body fat? The same number of calories consumed later in life would lead to swift obesity. (That doesn't seem fair.) The answer lies in the mysterious world of hormones, which work as messengers to tell your body what to do and when to accelerate the speed of metabolic reactions. Here are the main hormones involved in metabolism.

Let's look at Insulin-like Growth Factors. They come with pedigrees ranging from IGF 1 to IGF 8. These result from the breakdown of Human Growth Hormone. IGF stimulates cells to divide, enhancing rejuvenation of muscles, tissues and bone. As we age, HGH and IGF levels decline. A study by Dr. D. Rudman published in the *New England Journal of Medicine* in 1990 showed a link between HGH hormone levels and fat loss. The administration of Human Growth Hormone for six months was accompanied by an 8.8 percent increase in lean body mass, a 14.4 percent decrease in fat (adipose-tissue) mass, and a 1.6 percent increase in average lumbar vertebral bone mass[57]. The participants who were given HGH injections lost fat even though they did not diet or exercise. These findings give credence to the theory that HGH speeds metabolic reactions leading to the burning of fat.

Testosterone is the male hormone responsible for male attributes such as a lean, muscular body. Estrogen, a female hormone, can be found in men's bodies as well. (Incidentally, estrogen levels in men increase as they age, which counteracts the testosterone.) Some testosterone is found in women's bodies also. Blood concentration and a balance of sex hormones has been identified as playing a potential role in the regulation of fat distribution.

Women with upper-body obesity (as assessed using the waist-to-hip ratio) have a metabolic profile more similar to that of (apple shaped) men than of (pear shaped) women with lower-body obesity. These women have higher resting concentrations of free testosterone and lower concentrations of sex-hormone binding globulin[34,35,36,37]. Men with abdominal fat have low levels of free testosterone and Human Growth Hormone[35,36,74.]

The thyroid hormone is a major metabolic hormone. It regulates the body temperature by increasing or slowing down the speed of metabolic reactions that produce heat.

Insulin

After you eat, the glucose level in your blood rises, which triggers the pancreas to secrete insulin. Insulin opens glucose transport channels located on a cell's membranes. This is called insulin-stimulated glucose uptake and it's an important concept to those involved in dieting. The insulin causes a thirty-fold increase in the rate of glucose uptake by the body cells.

Insulin has anabolic action. It enables nutrients to enter cells and so provide building blocks necessary for protein synthesis. It is also one of the most important hormones in the weight-loss equation.

When the insulin level is high, glucose and fatty acids enter fat cells (adipose tissue) and are deposited as triacylglycerols (TG). In contrast, when there is no insulin in the blood, fatty acids can exit fat cells and are used as an energy source.

❖ ❖ ❖

What Is Fat?

Fat comprises molecules called triacylglycerol (TG), which are stored inside fat cells (adipocytes) as saturated fat. TG molecules are formed from fatty acids. These fatty acids are the product of digesting dietary fat — that fat in your rib-eye steak. That fact is the rationale behind the nutritionist's statement that "the fat you eat is the fat you wear." But you should also beware: the sugar water known as glucose can also be transformed into fatty acids.

Glycogen & Fat Storage

Now here is a concept that you must pay close attention to. Glycogen is the repository of glucose. In other words, sugar-water glucose is to glycogen what money is to a bank. In this case, we are talking branch banking. The liver and muscles are the major repository banks — holding places — for glycogen. Repeating this point: glucose collects in glycogen, which is deposited in two depositories: the Liver Bank and the Muscle Bank. Keeping that concept firmly in mind will help you to fully grasp how the CCD diet works.

Liver glycogen: The liver contains reserves of glycogen sufficient for an overnight fast. If you eat dinner at 7 p.m. and breakfast at 7 a.m., you have fasted 12 hours and the glycogen reserves in your liver have been depleted. Pouf, they are gone. That fast will become an important factor in your Calorie Cycling Diet. As you change from Steak Day to Baked Potato Day in your cycling diet, that 12 hour fast serves to deplete your liver glycogen. Keep that point in mind.

Muscle glycogen: Muscle glycogen, a larger form of stored carbs, provides instant energy to muscles. As molecules go, the glycogen molecule is extremely large. This has an important cosmetic effect for people with a large glycogen bankroll. The accumulation of big glycogen molecules in the muscles has a plumping effect that makes the muscles look larger[40].

If you are interested in how an Olympic sprinter calls up the emergency reserves of energy to win the gold medal, read on. Glycogen is a complex hydrated polymer of straight-chain glucose molecules. These form into a highly branched spherical structure. This highly branched spherical structure creates a large number of exposed terminal glucose molecules that are easily accessible to the enzymes involved in glycogen breakdown. That complex process is called glycogenolysis.

This ease of accessibility ensures an extremely rapid release of glucose molecules from glycogen during a fight-or-flight emergency situation, such as in a runner's final sprint[40]. In other words, this big glycogen molecule has the ability to break up into smaller glucose molecules that feed an intense amount of energy into the muscle tissues. Now you know how Seabiscuit, Secretariat and Smarty Jones won the Kentucky Derby.

- Glycogen Is a Repository for Glucose

❖ ❖ ❖

The Amazing Glycogen Molecule

Glycogen enables a muscle to generate a rapid release of energy. That capability is particularly important when the oxygen in the blood is insufficient to supply the body's instant demand for energy. This happens during periods of extremely vigorous muscle contraction — when exercise is performed at high intensity. If muscles suddenly need energy, such as during a 200-meter Olympic sprint, most of that energy called upon will be delivered from the anaerobic breakdown of muscle glycogen[40]. It's a runaround solution to a waning oxygen supply.

Chapter 2

Carbohydrate – Friend or Foe?

Carbohydrates make food sweet and satisfying, which is why we can eat them and easily shatter our daily calorie limit. In addition, carbs possess the highest insulin-invoking potential of any other food. As you have read, insulin is the blackest villain in making fat deposits.

Why are so many people addicted to refined carbohydrates? For one thing, carbs are an excellent source of instant energy. In the middle of the day when the concentration of our blood glucose drops, we need an energy boost, so we go for caffeine and a soft ice cream cone. Within minutes, this carb boost give us a sense of well being and satiety. But it also leads to a form of physical and psychological addiction. For just one day, try going without refined carbohydrates and you will experience an irresistible craving for a carb fix. Does the body crave them for nutritional value? No, refined carbohydrates have no nutritional value. We crave refined carbohydrates for the pleasant feeling they provoke, nothing more.

The Fat Machine

Many of us think that the deposition of fat takes place at the end of the day, when we go to sleep. That is the time when the body calculates the net in-and-out of calories, and puts the extra calories to one side. Well, folks, the body doesn't work that way. Research shows that most fat deposition happens in the first few minutes after eating refined carbohydrates. Refined carbs trigger insulin spike right away. That means fat deposition takes place at the point when the insulin level in your blood spikes. If there is too much glucose in the blood, insulin will force the glucose into body cells, including fat cells. The process is an ongoing balancing of energy that continues all day long. Fat deposition can happen at breakfast, lunch, dinner and snack time or any time when the glucose level is too high.

- The body does not perform calculations at the end of the day. It does not subtract the amount of calories burned from the amount of calories eaten and either store extra calories as fat, or extract them from fat. Rather, the balancing process is ongoing throughout the day. Remember, your body cannot see calories. It senses the amount of glucose in the blood.

The calories in the food you eat or the number of calories you use over a day is not the only factor that determines if you gain weight. Grossing out on a thousand calories of chocolate bar in two minutes will have a far worse impact than spreading consumption piece-by-piece throughout the day. The insulin spike in the first scenario will lead to instant fat deposition. If you eat the chocolate in small quantities, the calories will be used for energy and not end up on your rear end as fat. That is why it is important to eat small portions throughout the day, rather than three big meals. Keep that point always in mind.

The source of calories can also make a difference. If you eat a 200-calorie steak and a 200-calorie candy bar, the number of calories are the same, but the result in terms of fat storage is very different. The candy bar is more fattening because its glucose touches off that stormy insulin spike. Because of that difference, a concept called the glycemic index of food should be considered before you count calories.

The Glycemic Index

Not all carbs are alike. Some foods can have a relatively low amount of carbohydrates, but a high glycemic index. In that case, they make a poor choice for food. That's because even small amounts of high GI carbs touch off that stormy insulin secretion.

Using the glycemic index (GI) of carbohydrates empowers you to choose between the more fattening and less fattening carbs. Refined carbs digest faster and touch off a higher insulin spike. The more refined, the higher the spike. The body digests unrefined carbs more slowly. As a result the blood absorbs the glucose more gradually and insulin level rises slowly. The insulin level might not reach a threshold value because the blood glucose is burned for energy and consequently fat deposition might not occur. That kind of carbohydrate is said to have a low glycemic index.

Establishing glycemic index levels was simple. A sample group of a dozen or so healthy adults were tested for blood sugar level, which was recorded. The volunteers were then fed a sample serving of food — boiled rice, baked potato, jelly doughnut — and after a thirty minute wait for the blood sugar level to rise, they were tested again. The increases (spikes) in the blood sugar level were averaged and that figure became the GI for that food. For example, here are some carbohydrate foods and their GIs: white rice – 92; baked potato – 85; French fries – 75; macaroni and cheese — 64. Generally, you should choose carbs with GIs below 60. Examples include pasta, corn, peas, carrots, grapefruit, cherries, lentils, yogurt, nuts and pears.

The Bottom Line:

For a few days each week,

try to keep your insulin level low by

avoiding refined carbs

The goal of using the glycemic index is to bring your basal insulin level down to where it will not make you hungry, and will not force you to eat. So, if you are interested in good health and weight loss, follow this routine when choosing the foods you eat.

First, check the glycemic index; if it is more than 60, consider a food with a GI below 60.

Second, if the glycemic index is good, check the carbohydrate content. If it is high, consider another choice of food.

In summary, go for low GI and low grams of carbs.

❖ ❖ ❖

As discussed, you need not avoid all carbohydrates. Unprocessed carbohydrates should be included in your diet. Our bodies need them because carbohydrates:

* Provide an instant energy source especially for your muscles

Refined Carbs + Fat = Bad Deal

Because a rush of insulin allows nutrients to enter body cells, refined carbohydrates and fat are a bad food combination. Refined carbs initiate insulin secretion. Insulin opens the door and fat molecules — together with glucose — rush inside. The fat cell becomes bigger, and the next thing you know you need a bigger belt.

Remember

- Refined carbohydrates + fat = bad choice.

- Unprocessed carbohydrates + fat = okay

❖ ❖ ❖

Insulin Threshold Value

The rate that fat develops varies from person to person. That explains why your sleek, lithe friend seems able to eat more fattening foods than you can. Besides genetics, this happens for a number of reasons. There is a certain threshold level of insulin needed to open the door. If your body exceeds that amount, the glucose will enter the fat cells like water spilling over a ruptured dam. The threshold level differs from person to person. Also, the cells' responsiveness to insulin and anabolic hormone levels is also specific to each person.

As we age, our body's sensitivity to insulin changes. Each cell in our body carries insulin receptors. When someone gorges on refined carbs and produces a continually high level of insulin, these receptors stop reacting. Suddenly, the body becomes insulin resistant. Now comes Catch 22. Things become more acute because the insulin basal concentration in the blood adjusts and rises. As the insulin basal concentration elevates, we develop age-related insulin resistance. This creates a situation in which even a small elevation — even from a protein meal — causes an excess in the threshold concentration of insulin. Suddenly, glucose floods the fat cells like water over the dam.

What can we do about this unhealthy development? We need to bring the basal insulin concentration down. Taking a break from the carb overload we experience every day would be a first healthy step. Second, add regular exercise to our daily routine. Exercise weak up the muscles- it makes them metabolically active. Muscles consume calories as a sponge absorbs water.

Total Metabolism

To understand metabolism we should get to know its four elements: 1) basal metabolism, 2) exercise, 3) food and 4) temperature control. Let's look at each more closely.

Basal Metabolism: This is the minimum number of calories a resting body needs just to stay alive. This amounts to about 65 to 70 percent of total metabolism. As a rough gauge, some nutritionists say that basal metabolism burns about ten calories for each pound of weight. So a 135 pound person would burn 1,350 calories a day just to stay alive.

Exercise and Other Activity: This is the amount of calories burned during all activity during a 24-hour period. Exercise accounts for 15 to 25 percent of metabolism.

Heat Effect of Food: This is the increase in metabolism that takes place during the digestion and absorption of food. It accounts for 5 to 10 percent of total metabolism.

Adaptive Heat Generation: These are the calories used to produce body heat and keep body temperature regulated. It accounts for about 7 percent of total metabolism.

Here is how these elements work together. Basal metabolism (65 to 70 percent) + exercise (15 to 25 percent) + effect of food (5 to 10 percent) + temperature control (7 percent) = Total metabolism or Daily Calorie Needs (100 percent)

Thyroid Hormones and the Metabolic Rate

The thyroid gland regulates the metabolic rate. How does this work? A thyroid hormone, thyroxine, is created by combining the amino acid tyrosine with iodine. Thyroxine increases the number and activity of mitochondria in cells. Mitochondria is the energy producing unit of the cell. This increases energy production.

The administration of thyroid hormones such as thyroxine increases the rate of carbohydrate metabolism. It also accelerates the rate of protein synthesis and breakdown. Studies of obese women have shown that a certain percentage of women is suffering from an inactive, thyroid gland. When their thyroid levels were restored to normal with thyroid hormones, these women showed a significant fat loss[13].

Women should check their thyroid hormone level before initiating a fat-loss program. Thyroid hormone supplementation should be done only under a doctor's supervision since it carries a potential for overdosing. There is a safe way of stimulating thyroid gland function by supplementation with L-tyrosine and kelp. Please review the section on supplements in Part 2.

Chapter 3

The Calorie Cycling Diet

N

ow that you have a basic understanding of how metabolism works, the powerful role of hormones and the shattering impact of refined carbs, let's put it all together into a diet plan that will help you lose fat and build a lean body.

The Calorie Cycling Diet is so flexible that you can adjust it to any fitness need and lifestyle. The main advantage is it gives you the luxury of eating pleasurable food but in a controlled and managed way.

The Calorie Cycling Diet will protect you from the debilitating conditions of aging such as muscle loss, osteoporosis, as well as thickened artery walls (arteriosclerosis), diabetes, breast and colon cancer, stroke and heart attack (myocardial infarction). If you use this diet with an exercise program, the benefits will double, and you will add an extra element of anti-aging to it, rewarding you with more-active, disease-free years of life.

People who regularly exercise need fewer low-cal days than those who don't. Those who exercise can eat more carbs than those who don't.

- While this diet works best when combined with exercise, you can still benefit from it without exercising. Non-exercisers should be quite strict about refined carbohydrate consumption on low-cal days.

- Keep your insulin level low for most days of the week. In that way no fat deposition can take place.

As you learned, glycogen is stored in the muscles and the liver. The amounts are about 200 grams in the muscles and 70 grams in the liver. Muscle glycogen serves as an energy source for muscles and the liver's glycogen is used to maintain blood sugar at normal values. The liver's glycogen can be depleted — without exercise — by restricting carb intake for one day. Liver glycogen is the key to Calorie Cycling without doing exercises. During low-cal days the liver's glycogen becomes depleted. It restores on normal-cal days. Because the amount of glucose that can be stored in liver glycogen is smaller than that in muscle glycogen, be cautious about the amount of refined carbs you consume. You cannot gulp large amounts unless you exercise.

> You need to deplete your glycogen content
> before eating refined carbohydrates

On low-cal days you will eat mostly protein and get your energy from the amino acids in that steak. I recommend that you augment your diet with branched-chain amino acids in capsule form from Now Foods. Take a few capsules between each meal and at nighttime, whenever you feel hungry. The capsule form is convenient to carry on the go. You can use the supplement instead of the whey protein shake listed in the menus. (See Part 1, Chapter 4, Menus.) The branched-chain amino acids ward off hunger while providing essential amino acids.

Managing your food intake is an ongoing process. Some people practice this illogical philosophy: "Let me eat a cookie now, Later in the day, I will burn it off at the gym later." That's bum advice. First, you might not get to the gym. Second, and more important, fat is deposited as soon as you eat — not at the end of the day. By the time you get to the gym, the fat is cemented on as a new layer on your love handles. You must exercise hard to force the body to dig into those fat reserves.

There is a way to keep that cookie from turning into fat. Simply exercise before eating the cookie. Under these circumstances, the glucose from the cookie — if not used right away for energy — will enter muscle tissue or liver cells and be deposited there as glycogen,. That explains why Calorie Cycling is most effective when combined with an exercise program.

Let's look at this process a little more closely. When glucose enters the blood stream one of three things happen:

• First choice, it is used by body tissues for energy

• Second choice, it is deposited as glycogen in the liver and muscles if that depository is fully or partly depleted by exercise, and

• Third choice, it is deposited in fat cells (adipocytes), if there are no current energy needs.

The second point is all important in relation to the goals of this book. The liver glycogen serves as a major reserve for keeping the blood glucose level constant. In between meals, when there is no incoming glucose from food, the liver glycogen keeps blood glucose from falling dangerously low. The amount in the liver is just enough to get you through a 12-hour fast. When reserves of glycogen are depleted, the body starts to break down protein at an accelerated rate. This is how we lose valuable muscle tissue. It is the secret penalty lurking in the Atkins diet.

The amount of glycogen stored in muscles can vary. The larger the muscles, the more they can store. In other words, the storage capacity increases when your exercise builds bigger muscles. Muscle glycogen serves as a primary source of energy for as much as 20 minutes of intense exercise. Then muscle glycogen is depleted. The depletion of muscle glycogen is an important element of the Calorie Cycling process.

- The body will try to restore glycogen as soon as it has a chance. That means any carbohydrate you eat after exercise will be deposited as glycogen and not as fat

What it all means is that you can eat your favorite ice cream, cookies and pizza and not get fat. But, only under one condition.

- First, deplete your glycogen reserves

For glycogen depleting exercises, see Part 2.

To manage your diet, keep these six basic rules in a mind.

1. Do not eat refined carbohydrates and fat on the same day. Sweet, fat foods such as cake with frosting, cheese cake, regular ice cream and regular chocolate top the list of the most fattening foods. Sugar-free ice cream is fine.

2. If you are not exercising, do not drink more than 16 ounces of soda even on normal-cal days. Fructose does not provoke a big insulin spike. It is able to enter muscle cells and fat cells without the help of insulin. In other words, if you drink a soda, the fructose goes right to the cells and enters unhindered. If not used for energy, fructose can be converted to glucose. Natural fructose found in most fruits is fine because it is combined with fiber, which slows the rate of absorption. Both Coke and Pepsi are sweetened with commercial fructose.

3. Do not eat sweet desserts after meals. The sugar will make you hungry soon afterwards and make you crave more refined carbohydrates This is called "rebound" or "false" hunger.

4. When choosing foods, ask yourself, "Can I burn it off today?" and "What nutrients am I getting from this food?" If you cannot burn the energy or get nutrients from it, the food is not worth eating. Most of the time we eat because something tastes good — or to comfort ourselves — not because our body needs the nutrients. Consider the nutritional value in a sandwich. Bread gives you empty calories. The small amount of nutrients in lettuce and tomato has little value. Instead, why not eat a chicken breast with a salad? Choose foods that are rich in nutrients such as vegetables, soy products, beans, nuts, milk products, instead of those that lacking nutrients such as pasta, bread, bagels or pizza.

5. Do not eat large meals. Follow the ancient Japanese rule of *hara hachi-bu* (stop eating when you are 80 percent full). Become a grazer instead of a glutton. Spread your food consumption throughout the day — eat small amounts. Small portions keep insulin levels low. If you have a bowl of oatmeal for breakfast don't eat it all at once. Instead, eat half of it and snack on the rest between breakfast and lunch.

When eating frequently, be cautious. Research shows that people tend to consume more calories when they eat more than three times a day. It's a matter of habit. They keep eating the large portions that they have become accustomed to. Practice *hara hachi-bu*.

A Few Points on The Calorie Cycling Diet

The important rule: Do not start a normal-cal day if you honestly cannot say to yourself, "My previous day was calorie-restricted"

• On low-cal days, the only way you can lose fat is if you eat fewer calories than your body needs (Negative Calorie Balance)

• Do not become disappointed if you fail to resist cravings. Given time, the hunger and cravings will ease.

• For those who are already exercising, you might want to start with 1-3 regimen.

• On low-cal days, eat all the green vegetables you like.

• If you want fast results, limit your fat consumption to no more than 50 grams a day on low-cal days. Consider that there are hidden fat in food that you eat. Supplement with Omega 3-6-9 oil 5-10 g per day.

Cycling Regimens

The Cal Cycling Diet lets you lose fat and build a lean body because it alternates catabolism (food breakdown) with anabolism (tissue building). As soon as you became accustomed to the cycling pattern, you can adjust your level of calorie consumption to suit your needs. If you feel you need more energy for exercising, do one of two things: 1) increase the amount of carbs in your diet or 2) temporary lower the number of low-cal days in your regimen. If you feel you need to lose fat, do the opposite for a week or two. With The Calorie Cycling Diet, you can eat all of your favorite foods — within moderation — and by adjusting the diet, you can maintain your weight, lose fat, or build muscles. It's up to you.

The Calorie Cycling plan varies according to each person's activity level and objectives.

Calorie Cycling starts with a 1-1 regimen (one day of normal calories and one of lower calories) and can be extended to 1-6. The first number signifies normal-cal days. The second number stands for the number of days calories are restricted. The cycling regimen can be anywhere changed from 1-1 to 1-6. The 1-6 regimen is one day on a normal-cal day and six days on a low-cal diet.

Later in the book I will show macro-cycling regimens when number of normal-cal days is extended. These types of regimens are useful for those who are interested in building muscles.

In Table 1, a 1-1 regimen is shown.

Table 1 Cycling regimens

1-1

Mon	Tue	Wed	Thurs	Fri	Sat	Sun
Catabolism	Anabolism	Catabolism	Anabolism	Catabolism	Anabolism	Catabolism
Low Cal	Normal Cal	Low Cal	Normal Cal	Low Cal	Normal Cal	Low Cal
Exercise	Strength training	Aerobic exercise	Strength training	Aerobic exercise	Strength training	OFF

This diet offers a subset of levels, a neat way to manage the amount of calories you consume on low-cal days. The three levels are

- Level A (50-75 % of Daily Calorie Needs) is for beginners.

- Level B (50% of Daily Calorie Needs)

Novices may wish to start with a 1-1 cycle at Level A and proceed to Levels B while staying with the 1-1 sequence. After that you can increase the number of low-cal days to 1-2 and so on.

Here are examples of 1-2, 1-3, and 1-4:

1-2

Mon	Tue	Wed	Thurs	Fri	Sat	Sun	Mon
Anabolism	Cat	Cat	Anabolism	Cat	Cat	Anabolism	Cat
Cal	Low	Low	Normal Cal	Low	Low	Normal Cal	Low

1-3

Mon	Tue	Wed	Thurs	Fri	Sat	Sun	Mon
Anabolism	Cat	Cat	Cat	Anabolism	Cat	Cat	Cat
Cal	Low	Low	Low	Normal Cal	Low	Low	Low

1-4

Mon	Tue	Wed	Thurs	Fri	Sat	Sun	Mon
Anabolism	Cat	Cat	Cat	Cat	Anabolism	Cat	Cat
Cal	Low	Low	Low	Low	Normal Cal	Low	Low

Eating on a Normal-cal Day

A normal-cal day should feel like a normal eating day with sweet desserts allowed. You may eat approximately 350 to 400 grams of carbohydrates on a normal-cal day. This is the typical amount of carbohydrates in the average adult's daily diet. You can consume up to 90 g of fat on these days.

If you are not exercising, don't over-partake of the generous carb allowance by stuffing yourself with cookies, cake and pie. When choosing your menu, eat foods that give you a sense of satiety. Boiled potatoes rate quite high on the satiety index of fullness. High sugar foods have a low satiety index and stimulate cravings for more sugary foods. High-fat foods like cheesecake also rate badly. Foods with moderate amounts of fat, such as lean steak, rate excellent.

Here are other examples of the satiety (satisfaction) index range:

- Cakes, doughnuts and cookies are among the least filling

- When choosing fruit, oranges and apples outscore bananas

- Fish is more satisfying than lean beef or chicken

- Popcorn is twice as filling as a candy bar or peanuts

Table 2 Satiety index

[Avoid foods with low satiety (satisfaction) numbers.]

Potatoes	320
Fish	220
Oatmeal	210

Oranges	200
Apples	195
Brown pasta	190
Beef	175
Baked beans	170
Whole grain bread	160
Grapes	160
Popcorn	155
All Bran	150
Grain bread	150
Eggs	150
Cheese	145
White rice	135
Honey snacks	130
Brown Rice	130
Lentils	130
Crackers	125
Cookies	120
White pasta	120
Bananas	120
Corn flakes	115
Special K	115
French fries	115
Muesli	100

White bread	100
Ice cream	95
Crisps	90
Peanuts	85
Yogurt	85
Mars bar	70
Cake	65
Croissant	45

While all carbohydrates are allowed on a normal-cal day, here are some general recommendations. After noon, avoid refined carbohydrates unless you are coming off an exercise session. In other words, no Wonder Bread after lunch — unless you pump iron.

For those who exercise, the best time to eat refined carbohydrates is within a two-hour period after the exercise. Those who want to build muscles should consume some protein along with the carbs — in a ratio of one part protein to four parts of carbohydrate. Whey Protein Shake with carbs is a best choice.

Tip: Choose carbohydrates that contain fiber instead of refined carbohydrates. The glycemic index will help you to make right choices.

Eating on a Cal-Restricted Day

Initially, low-cal days will pose the biggest challenge. In the beginning, do not eat foods containing sugar or white flour such as candy, cookies, white bread and bagels. During the first two weeks, your total carbohydrate intake on low-cal days should be no more than 150 grams a day. That's about 25 grams of carbs during each of six meals. Try to limit consumption of fat to 50 g (Omega oils are included in this number).

Keep the following levels in mind to guide you on low-cal days.

Level A

50-75 % of Daily Calorie Needs

Level B

50 % of Daily Calorie Needs (DCN)

Remember to start The Calorie Cycling Diet slowly. Do not jump to a high level of restriction. Start with Level A. Do this in the right way, otherwise you might become disappointed if you fail to stick to the regimen and fall short in managing your craving for food.

Here are some suggestions to assure success on low-cal days:

• Make a list of your favorite snacks. Put those you cannot live without at the top of your list.

• Remove temptation by removing from your home the refined carbohydrates that you crave. Instead, keep sugar-free snacks available (f. e. Jell-o)

• In the beginning, keep a diary and make entries at each meal.

A Word to the Wise:
Cold Turkey Is Better than Just One Bite

When it comes to avoiding refined carbohydrates, many of us face the temptation to have just one bite to satisfy a craving. This doesn't work and never will. Here's why.

As soon as you eat even a small quantity of refined carbohydrates — French fries, chocolate cake — your insulin spikes for a few minutes. After the insulin pushes the glucose into your cells, the blood glucose level drops. Crash. This causes your body to crave more refined carbohydrates. The cycle continues and eating refined carbs becomes an uncontrollable behavior, invoking a Catch 22 chain reaction.

❖ ❖ ❖

Chapter 4

Sample Menus

The following menus are example of what you might have on a 1-1 regimen.

Monday: a Low-Cal Day

Your menu on low-cal days consists mostly of protein. While protein itself does not reduce body fat, it does keeps you from getting hungry while providing relatively small amount of calories. You will lose fat because you have a negative calorie balance as a result of eating a protein-rich diet. If you eat a lot of fat on this day, you will not lose fat. In this case calories are calories, no matter where they come from. (There are situations where calories are not calories. Remember the 200 calories from steak compared to the same amount from ice cream?)

Mind you now, don't eliminate all fats. On low-cal days, you should consume healthy fat such as Omega-3, Omega-6 and Omega-9. The best source is fish oil, which you can buy in a health food store. Do not try to save money by choosing on low price. Almost all fish — especially those from fish farms — are contaminated these days with heavy metals, mercury and PCBs. That's not good for young people and young mothers. The fish oil should be detoxified, but not all companies do that. The trusted brands are Health from the Sun, and Now Foods. You should consume at least 2.5 grams a day.

Leave a table feeling not hungry but not satiated. Japanese parents admonish their children to leave the table before their stomachs feel full. Indeed, it has been proven in repeated studies that a slight daily calorie-deficiency contributes to long life.

9 a.m. — Breakfast

Feta cheese omelet

Coffee with whole milk and Splenda or Nutrasweet

11 a.m. — Optional Snack

Whey protein shake or egg whites / branched chain amino acids (3 capsules)

Noon — First Lunch

Beef or chicken soup

2 p.m. — Second lunch

Salmon with vegetable salad with olive or safflower oil dressing

5 p.m. — Optional Snack

Whey protein shake or egg whites / branched chain amino acids (3 capsules)

6 p.m. — Dinner

Turkey breast with green salad

9 p.m. — Snack

Whey protein shake or egg whites / branched chain amino acids (3 capsules)

Tips for Managing Hunger

Boil a dozen eggs; separate the whites from the yolks and keep the whites in the refrigerator. When hunger strikes, eat some for a quick pick-me-up.

Have a Whey Protein shake in the refrigerator. Drink it between meals.

Snack on nuts, which have a good balance of healthy oils.

Tuesday: a Normal-Cal Day

Eat as you normally would eat today, but keep this tip in mind:

Watch your calorie consumption.

 Do not overeat unless exercised intensively.

9 a.m. — Breakfast

Pancakes with jam, or cereal with milk or bagel with cream cheese

Coffee with the one percent milk

Noon — First Lunch

Three bean soup

2 p.m. — Second Lunch

Pasta with cheese and sauce

6 p.m. — Dinner

Steak with fried potatoes

7 p.m. – Snack

Cup of ice cream

Wednesday: a Low-Cal Day

9 a.m. — Breakfast

2 sausages, spinach omelet

Coffee with whole milk, Splenda or Nutrasweet

11 a.m. — Optional Snack

Whey protein shake or egg whites / branched chain amino acids (3 capsules)

Noon — First Lunch

Italian wedding soup

2 p.m. — Second lunch

Chicken grilled with pieces of orange, vegetable salad

5 p.m. — Optional Snack

Whey protein shake or egg whites / branched chain amino acids (3 capsules)

6 p.m. — Dinner

Pork chops with green salad

9 p.m. — Snack

Whey protein shake or egg whites / branched chain amino acids (3 capsules)

Thursday: a Normal-Cal Day

9 a.m. — Breakfast

Bagel with cream cheese

Coffee with the 1 percent milk

Noon — First Lunch

Vegetable soup

2 p.m. — Second Lunch

Slice of pizza

6 p.m. — Dinner

Steak with mashed potatoes

7 p.m. – Snack

Cup of low-fat yogurt

Friday: a Low-Cal Day

9 a.m. — Breakfast

Ground beef hamburger (no bread or bun)

Coffee with whole milk, Splenda or Nutrasweet

11 a.m. — Optional Snack

Whey protein shake or egg whites / branched chain amino acids (3 capsules)

Noon — First Lunch

Grilled chicken salad with olive or safflower oil dressing

2 p.m. — Second lunch

2 boiled eggs with mayonnaise

5 p.m. — Optional Snack

Whey protein shake or egg whites / branched chain amino acids (3 capsules)

6 p.m. — Dinner

Stuffed pepper with sour cream

9 p.m. — Snack

Whey protein shake or egg whites / branched chain amino acids (3 capsules)

Saturday: a Normal-Cal Day

9 a.m. — Breakfast

Bowl of cereal with 1 percent milk

Coffee with 1 percent milk

Noon — First Lunch

Bowl of fruit with whipped cream

2 p.m. — Second Lunch

Pasta with cheese and sauce

6 p.m. — Dinner

Turkey breast with boiled broccoli

Sunday: a Low-Cal Day

9 a.m. — Breakfast

Mushroom and onion omelet

Coffee with whole milk, Splenda or Nutrasweet

11 a.m. — Optional Snack

Whey protein shake or egg whites / branched chain amino acids (3 capsules)

Noon — First Lunch

Grilled chicken with green salad (w/olive or safflower oil dressing)

2 p.m. — Second lunch

Fish with a vegetable salad

5 p.m. — Optional Snack

Whey protein shake or egg whites / branched chain amino acids (3 capsules)

6 p.m. — Dinner

Pork chops w/vegetables

9 p.m. — Snack

Whey protein shake or egg whites / branched chain amino acids (3 capsules)

✤ ✤ ✤

How to Cycle Your Daily Diet

Start with a 1-1 regimen and gain experience at managing your cravings for refined carbohydrates. After a few weeks, you can progress to a 1-2 regimen: one normal-cal day followed by two low-cal days, one normal-cal day followed by two low-cal days, and so on.

The 1-1 regimen is meant to introduce you to Calorie Cycling. It is not an effective regimen since people who are not accustomed to managing cravings tend to fail on low-cal days.

Note: If you are not exercising, follow at least a 1-4 regimen (one normal-cal day followed by four low-cal days.)

1-2 or 1-3 regimen is not effective for those who are not exercising.

Coping with Sweet Cravings

Here are some tips to help you resist cravings on low-cal days:

• Tell yourself, "I can eat this doughnut tomorrow. Today, I must avoid it."

• Have a whey protein isolate from Now Foods. You can buy it at any health food store. Compared to other whey proteins, this brand has no carbohydrates and it tastes better. You may drink some anytime during the day. Enjoy this drink; there is no limit to the amount you may have. Please refer to Part 3 for the recipe for the protein shake.

• Even if you are not hungry, eat small amounts of protein — beef, chicken, pork, tofu or egg whites (up to dozen a day) — every two hours. This will prevent hunger and stop a craving before it hits you. Use this preventive tactic.

- Have a sugar-free "cheat" snack when a craving hits. These include sugar-free hot chocolate, sugar-free ice cream.

- Have fruit instead of refined carbohydrates if you cannot resist a craving. Fructose from fruit will not cause a chain reaction because it does not call up a spike in insulin secretion.

For the first few months, you will find it difficult to control your cravings for refined carbohydrates because your basal insulin level is elevated. Your pancreas, which is accustomed to secreting high amounts of insulin, takes a few months to lower it. Then your cravings will become manageable.

To kill your cravings on a low-cal day, use supplements. After 6 p.m., use Gymnema Sylvestre (two capsules) together with Garcinia Cambogia (two capsules) and liquid L–Carnitine (2 to 6 tablespoons) to prevent sweet cravings at night. These herbs are non-stimulants. They will not keep you awake and they are safe to use for long-term use. Take them daily for the first two months to help you get accustomed to your eating pattern. (For more information, see the section on supplements in Part 2.)

Given time, you will adjust to the new eating schedule while you learn your weak points and how to prevent cravings. In the end, it will make a difference — giving you control over your body and the ability to control your weight.

Making Adjustments

After six weeks, if you do not see the weight loss results you seek, get a bit more serious about restricting your calorie intake. If that step does not work, increase the number of low-cal days in your regimen. You can temporarily switch to a 1-6 regimen, then go back to 1-2 or 1-3. You see, the CCD diet really is flexible.

There will be times when you might break your schedule. If you skip your daily exercise, make the day low-cal day, at Level B (50 % of DCN): protein and green vegetables. That should get you back on track.

The Most Common Mistake

The mistake that people make most often is to starve on low-cal days and binge on normal-cal days.

Tips for Success

Make sure you don't feel hunger on low-cal days. Consume a whey protein drinks as much as possible.

Eat normally on normal-cal days. That doesn't mean you can stuff yourself with all those cupcakes you missed on low-cal days.

While Calorie Cycling prevents your metabolism from catabolic dominance, the following measure will help to boost anabolism and increase your total metabolism.

Exercising

Countless studies show that exercise increases the secretion of anabolic hormones regardless of your age. Part 2 will describe the role of exercise.

✿ ✿ ✿

Part 2

Your Guide to Exercise

- How to perform exercises to burn glycogen
- Achieve results with minimum efforts
- Save money by not buying useless supplements

Chapter 5

Exercise and Intensity

Many studies have demonstrated that vigorous exercise increases levels of Human Growth Hormone and testosterone in the blood[16,17,24]. The more hormones in your blood, the better your body works. Hormones make for better cognition, energy, sex and skin. As well, it has been shown that exercise prevents some forms of cancer (breast and gastrointestinal), improves blood pressure control and the blood lipid profile. It also prevents arteriosclerosis, insult and myocardial infarction[2]. The list can go on. Consider the anabolic hormones as your defensive shield. It protects against diseases and aging. During history, nature predisposed us to be physically active. If your heart is not forced to pump blood at an accelerated rate, you are one step closer to being dead. Running is our natural state of being. Anything less is unhealthy and leaves us disease prone. Make a move; take the first step. Even a small step is better than none. Do it regularly. Impulsive exercising is not effective and is dangerous.

Exercise can be performed in many ways. Slow. Fast. With light weights or heavy. Doing small number of repetitions with heavy weight or a high number with lighter weight. Rest between activities or keep moving. So many options. Depending on your goal, you can find one that suits you. But keep in a mind : Your body is highly adaptive. It can adjust to exercise and even then it will find a way to conserve energy.

At some point, you can expect to stop losing fat or building muscle mass. Chalk it up to the body's ability to adapt to new lifestyle patterns. Solution? Fool your body. Alternate your physical activities. Change the physical stress that you apply on your body.

Exercise and carbohydrate restriction go hand in hand. The more exercise you get, the less restrictive your diet regimen needs to be. In other words, if you want to eat more of your favorite cake, add more exercise into your Calorie Cycling Diet. For sedentary couch potatoes, the recommended cycling regimen is 1-6 at Level B. That means one normal-cal day, followed by six low-cal days, at Level B. For an alert and active person who gets regular and intense exercise, the cycling regimen is less strict, a 1-3 at Level A, or one normal-cal day to three low-cal days. So, the more frequent and intense your exercise, the freer you are to dine high on the hog.

Eat your carbohydrates after exercising. After you exercise, you may notice a carbohydrate craving. This is a normal reaction because your body is urgently trying to restore its glycogen supply, which can take up to 12 hours. During first 4 hours you can eat refined carbohydrates without worrying about increases in fat.

How much food can you eat? Gram for gram, no direct correlation can be made between glycogen and carbohydrate. Rather, the size of glycogen reserves depends mostly on individual muscle mass, which is why the amount you can eat following exercise will differ from person to person. It's something you will have to learn from your body.

There may be times when you need a pre-exercise carbohydrate. Do you ever lack the energy to go to the gym because you have been on a diet? Research shows that carbohydrate restriction before exercise is associated with early onset of fatigue during physical exercise[15,25,30].

Before and during exercise, you may consume fructose and caffeine in the form of sports drinks. That should provide a jolt needed to keep going through a workout[21]. (One such drink is called Extreme Energy Shot made by Arizona). I recommend fructose instead of other sugars because it provides energy without provoking a large insulin secretion. Studies have shown that insulin blocks the release of exercise-induced Human Growth Hormone.

Post-Workout Calorie Burn

Studies of athletes have shown that the more intense the exercise, the longer the post-workout impact on metabolism and calorie burning[7,16,17]. In other words, after intense exercise, you continue to burn calories at accelerated rate for a few hours. Intensive weight lifting has a greater impact on post-workout calorie burn than aerobic running or swimming. That is one of many reasons why intensive weight lifting is important part of Calorie Cycling exercise program. Active muscles, speaking metamorphically, consume calories as a sponge absorbs water.

✧ ✧ ✧

Aerobic Exercise

Aerobic refers to oxygen available in the tissues for generating energy. Examples of aerobic exercises are running and swimming to condition the heart and lungs. The process of energy generation can be either aerobic (using oxygen) or anaerobic (without oxygen). When the level of intensity rises the muscles start to generate energy anaerobically. Have you ever felt a "Second wing"? That is a moment when anaerobic energy generation starts to dominate over aerobic.

Any exercise performed at less than 65 percent of maximum effort is considered as aerobic.

Examples of aerobic exercise:

• Running below 65 percent of maximum effort

• Weight lifting at low intensity

The benefits of aerobic exercise include:

• Increased tissue sensitivity to insulin[23]

• Fat is burned as a primary energy source

• Strengthened heart and lungs, which improves blood circulation and delivers more nutrients to the tissues

• Improved blood circulation in the kidneys and tissues -actions that remove toxic metabolites (detoxification action)

• Improved blood circulation, which delivers more oxygen and nutrients to every cell in your body (improving cell's functions)

Anaerobic Exercise

Anaerobic production of energy can be used in emergency situations when a large amount of energy is needed, but there is not enough oxygen to generate it. Any exercise performed at high intensity, close to maximum effort would be anaerobic.

Anaerobic exercise usually refers to weight lifting because this type of exercise involves bursts of power when the energy need is extreme. Running can be anaerobic if it is performed intensely, during sprinting, for example.

The benefits of anaerobic exercise include:

- Increased anabolic hormone secretions[16,17,24]

- Efficiently depletes muscle glycogen — important for losing fat

- A long post-workout calorie-burning benefit

- Production of a large amount of lactic acid — a natural antioxidant

Improves strength of bones and ligaments

Increases turnover of Ca in bones

Increases muscle strength and mass

Given this information, one might wonder: Which type of exercise should I be doing to lose the most fat? Aerobic or anaerobic?

Each type of exercise has specific health benefits. The best course of action would be to alternate the days of aerobic exercises with those of anaerobic exercises.

The Calorie Cycling Diet recommends performing both aerobic and anaerobic exercises in a balanced matter. Each individual should have his own number of aerobic (low-cal) and anaerobic (normal-cal) days in the regimen. This customization depends on individual's genetic abilities and can be detected by testing DNA for polymorphisms.

Why emphasize the importance of exercise? Because it is the only way to stay energetic, fit and disease free. It's the best way to add 10 to 20 additional years to your life. If you calculate the time spent exercising, it should almost equal the time you add to your life.

- High Intensity: It Brings Results.

- It Invokes Anabolic Hormone Release.

Intensity in a workout puts stress on your muscles and your whole body. Let's look at that more closely. The amount of work your muscles perform in a minute depends on the intensity level. In running, it correlates with your running speed. The faster your run, the greater the intensity — and the more calories you burn. When you lift weights, the heavier the weights, the greater the effort. That translates as more stress on your body. In response, the stressed body releases Human Growth Hormone and testosterone[16,17,24] to help fight the stress. Low intensity exercise does not produce this effect.

While keeping in mind that any exercise is better than none, exercise should be efficient. Otherwise, why exercise? What makes it efficient? High intensity. Why is exercise at high intensity important? High intensity achieves four major benefits:

- It allows you to cut exercise time because it burns a large amount of calories in the least amount of time

- It conditions your body. In other words, it trains it

- It depletes muscle glycogen — very important.

- It stimulates Human Growth Hormone and testosterone release

Twenty minutes of intense exercise can deplete your muscle glycogen content to where the fat-producing carbohydrates you consume afterwards will not deposit glucose in fat cells. Instead, they will be converted to glycogen. Any person exercising should try to achieve high intensity workouts, but the rule you should follow is this:

- Start easy and slow. Over time work your way to a high intensity level.

- Warm up and stretch before each exercise session.

If your goal is to build muscles, you should follow this basic principle of weight lifting: The optimum workout time is between 55 and 80 minutes.

To build muscles, you need to achieve the following:

• A level of muscle stress that tears the muscle fibers (myofibrils) When the torn myofibrils knit back together, the new bonds are bigger and tighter and the muscles grow in size.

• A high level of desirable anabolic hormones in the blood

• An abundance of protein and other nutrients

• Be in a Positive Calorie Balance

Before the myofibril muscle fibers can be torn, a certain level of load must be placed on the muscle. When you are young, you can tolerate this kind of intensity and load in a workout. But as you age, it is harder to reach this level. You tire easier than you did at age 20.What can you do to raise the intensity to higher levels? You can use energy producing supplements immediately before workouts. One of them is Creatine Monohydrate. See Sports Supplements for a list.

Consider these training options. High intensity, vigorous exercise triggers the release of Human Growth Hormone and testosterone. The higher the level of the hormones, the better because they stimulate sagging metabolism. From this perspective, alternating periods of speed acceleration with periods of slower activity is a beneficial way to train.

Option 1: For a running exercise, I recommend accelerating four times during a 20-minute run. For each acceleration, run two minutes at 55 to 80 percent of your maximum speed. Then slow down and continue to run at slower pace.

Option 2: Interval training — work and rest — is also beneficial, especially for beginners.

Option 3: You can split your exercise session into two parts, with rest in between. In this case, increase the speed you run during each part of session. For example, instead of running 30 minutes at 6.1 mph run twice, 15 minutes each time at 7.3 mph.

Option 4: Here is an example of interval training that I developed for my clients. I call it **Manhattan Rush**:

Set a treadmill on 2% incline and 4.8 mph speed.

Start walking very fast--almost run. Your arms should move as during running. Do it for 30 seconds.

Start running without changing treadmill's speed. Try to relax and rest while running. Do it for 30 seconds.

Return to fast walking without changing treadmill's speed.

Continue 30 sec - 30 sec pattern for 15 minutes.

Run the last 5-10 minutes.

Note that you can reverse the order in start your exercise with running for 10 minutes and then switch to walk-run pattern.

This **Manhattan Rush** exercise is good as for beginners as well as for experienced fitness enthusiasts. It helps to diminish fat in thighs, hip, abdominal area and buttocks.

Advise: use elastic shorts for cyclists – it helps to avoid irritation between the legs.

Deprivation Diets Simply Don't Work

Ask a group of athletes if they can perform their best while they are being denied carbohydrates. They'll laugh at you. When it comes to physical activities, carbohydrates are essential energy sources.

This is why the "eat less, exercise more" concept, if taken blindly, can actually work against you, especially as you age. First of all, your body needs more nutrients and more calories when you start an exercise program to effectively repair any micro-traumas, especially in joints and muscles. Prolonged calories or food restriction leads to nutritional deficiencies. Secondly, studies show that people lose protein (muscles) even while exercising on calorie-restricted diets.

Thirdly, a high volume of exercise on calorie-restricted diets suppresses the release of anabolic hormones, slows down your metabolism and leads to overtraining. Overtraining is a metabolic condition resulted from excessive exercise without adequate periods of rest. Rest days are important component of the Calorie Cycling Diet exercise program. If at any time you feel tired or sleepy, lose interest in exercise, or perform worse, you are probably on the edge of overtraining; take a week of rest. Here is example of how the rest days can be included into your program:

Table 1-1 Cycling regimens

1-1

Mon	Tue	Wed	Thurs	Fri	Sat	Sun
Catabolism	Anabolism	Catabolism	Anabolism	Catabolism	Anabolism	Catabolism
Low Cal	Normal Cal	Low Cal	Normal Cal	Low Cal	Normal Cal	Low Cal
Exercise	Strength training	OFF	Strength training	OFF	Strength training	OFF

MAX Effort - A Special Exercise to Increase Your Metabolism

You have learned that to increase metabolism, you need to make sure that you consume your daily calorie needs. But you can do more. Besides consuming enough calories, you can perform anabolic hormone releasing exercises (MAX Effort exercises). It takes only 20 minutes a day, but is the most effective way to boost HGH and testosterone production. Dozens of studies have shown that a burst of power during heavy weight lifting leads to an increase in blood HGH and testosterone concentration.

Caution: this type of exercise is not for everyone. Only absolutely healthy individuals who have previous experience with heavy weight lifting should be doing it. If you are not customized with a heavy weight lifting, start with moderate weight and progress gradually over a period of 12 to 24 months. Recent studies also show that a burst of heavy exercise performed by untrained individuals can invoke heart attack, blood vessels rupture, stroke or even eye damage! So be cautious!

The MAX Effort exercise can be done as a bench press or a leg press. It can also be performed as a deadlift or barbell squat, but only by experienced weight lifters since if done incorrectly, it may cause severe injuries. Before starting this exercises review machine instructions and consult a personal trainer for proper technique!

How to perform the MAX Effort bench press:

Use the Smith machine. It has safety hooks that eliminate the need for a spotter. The Nautilus press machine can be used also.

Caution: Do not perform this exercise with a free bar without a spotter! Always warm up with a few sets using medium weight.

Set a slight angle on the bench.

Find your 1 RM (1 Repetition Maximum).

3. Deduct 30 pounds from 1 RM weight.

4. Do 8 sets of 3 repetitions.

That's it. You're done. It should take you only 15-20 minutes to complete this exercise. Stay with 3 reps for a while (a month or two) before moving to 2 reps and increasing the weight. I do not recommend 1 rep since it may cause injuries. Check your 1 RM once a week.

This type of exercise is meant to increase anabolic hormone release. If performed properly it provides significant anti-aging benefits. You will start feeling more energetic, especially at the end of the day. The effect may last for up to two days. Review your exercise program if you do not feel increase in energy level. You may be doing too much exercising with little amount of rest days that restrains the anabolic hormones release. Take a few days off.

Do not train too hard on this day. It may reverse anabolism into catabolism, the opposite of what we are looking for. Exercise, if performed intensively, leads to a post-exercise catabolic state. Cortisol is released as a result of the physical stress. This is one of the reasons why I recommend consuming carbohydrate-heavy meals right after weight lifting session – to stop cortisol release and prevent catabolism.

Chapter 6

Glycogen-Depleting Resistance Training

An intensive 20-minute exercise will deplete glycogen. Many people find it is difficult to maintain this high level of exercise intensity. An alternative way to exercise is to keep your muscles under moderate tension as long as possible because that depletes glycogen quickly and without Herculean effort. It is easy to do on any resistance machine such as Bowflex or Crossbow or similar equipment found in a gym. You can use moderate weights as well. Women can easily perform this exercise. For them, it is a preferable technique for weight training because it does not require great muscle strength. It also saves time, A person can be in and out of gym within 30 minutes with a complete body workout.

Method

Choose a low-to-moderate resistance or weight. Exercise the biggest muscles first: chest and legs. Do the following:

Take the Chest Fly position (pectorals). Lie on an inclined bench. Extend your arms fully. Grasp low handles with palms facing up and arms at shoulder level. Keep elbows slightly bent, pull the handles together over the chest in a hugging motion. Stop your arms halfway together (45-degree angle) and hold it in this position until your muscles fail. Breathe deeply. Do not hold your breath. Repeat three to four times.

1. Switch to the leg press position (quadriceps).

2. Push a medium weight and hold it in a half way through until your muscles fail. Repeat a few times.

3. Rotate to other muscle groups.

Note: You will experience muscle ache while performing this type of exercise. This means your muscle tissues are accumulating lactic acid, a result of glycogen breakdown. Hold on as long as you can. You can do slight flexions and extensions with small amplitude while holding. The muscles should stay tense. Do not relax them between each repetition.

The physiology of this method is twofold.

• It forces muscles to deplete local glycogen. Muscle tension cuts off the blood supply to the tissues, so blood glucose cannot be delivered for replacement energy.

• It burns the largest number of calories in the briefest period of time.

This type of exercise is very helpful when training back muscles on Roman chair. Just stay in one position as long as you can or do very slight movements. This kind of exercise prevents spine injuries and good for those who had a slip disk in the past.

❖ ❖ ❖

When combining diet and exercise, some people find the following schedules useful.

1-1

	Mon	Tues	Wed	Thu	Fri	Sat	Sun
Exercise	Strength training 60 min	Aerobic 60 min	Strength training 60 min	Aerobic 60 min	Strength training 60 min	Off	Off
Diet	Normal Cal	Low Cal	Normal Cal	Low Cal	Normal Cal	Low Cal	Low Cal

1-2

	Mon	Tues	Wed	Thu	Fri	Sat	Sun
Exercise	Strength training 60 min	Aerobic 60 min	Aerobic 60 min	Strength training 60 min	Aerobic 60 min	Aerobic 60 min	Off
Diet	Normal Cal	Low Cal	Low Cal	Normal Cal	Low Cal	Low Cal	Low Cal

1-3

	Mon	Tues	Wed	Thurs	Fri	Sat	Sun
Exercise	Strength training 60 min	Aerobic 60 min	Aerobic 60 min	Aerobic 60 min	Strength training 60 min	Aerobic 60 min	Off
Diet	Normal Cal	Low Cal	Low Cal	Low Cal	Normal Cal	Low Cal	Low Cal

Do your strength training/weight lifting on normal-cal days!

If you exercise regularly you need to have carbohydrates in your diet since they are important source of energy, but you need to be careful. Too much of it can cause fat deposition.

Question: Can I mix circuit training with other forms of aerobic exercises during one exercise session?

Answer: Absolutely! In fact, I urge you to mix aerobic exercises in order to fire up as many muscles as possible.

From Micro-cycling to Macro-cycling: From Losing Fat to Building Muscles

The regimens described above are described as Micro-cycling — there are few normal-cal days in the cycle. Micro-cycling promotes fat loss. When the number of normal-cal days exceeds two, the regimen becomes Macro-cycling — there are several normal-cal days in the cycle. These regimens are used to build muscle. If at any time you detect that your muscles are becoming atrophic or you need to give your body a better nutritional jolt, there is a solution: Switch to Macro-cycling, It puts you in anabolic predominance needed to build muscles. The regimens start from 2–2 and can be extended up to 14–7 or 14-14.

For those who concentrate on building muscles, the following regimens can be used:

2-2

	Mon	Tues	Wed	Thu	Fri	Sat	Sun
Exercise	Weight Lifting Upper body 60 min	Weight Lifting Lower body 60 min	Aerobic 60 min	Aerobic 60 min	Weight Lifting Upper body 60 min	Weight Lifting Lower body 60 min	Off
Diet	Normal Cal	Normal Cal	Low Cal	Low Cal	Normal Cal	Normal Cal	Low Cal

People usually start with upper body exercise, followed by lower body exercise, but it really doesn't matter which is first. What is important is to work out the muscles really hard, to actually damage them on the cellular level, so that new protein tissue can grow. Most people just exercise — making their muscles work — which is not enough stimuli to make them grow.

2-3

	Mon	Tues	Wed	Thu	Fri	Sat	Sun
Exercise	Weight Lifting Upper body 60 min	Weight Lifting Lower body 60 min	Off	Aerobic 60 min	Aerobic 60 min	Weight Lifting Upper body 60 min	Weight Lifting Lower body 60 min
Diet	Normal Cal	Normal Cal	Low Cal	Low Cal	Low Cal	Normal Cal	Normal Cal

2-5

	Mon	Tues	Wed	Thu	Fri	Sat	Sun
Exercise	Off	Circuit training 60 min	Off	Aerobic 60 min	Aerobic 60 min	Weight Lifting Upper body 60 min	Weight Lifting Lower body 60 min
Diet	Low Cal	Low Cal	Low Cal	Low Cal	Low Cal	Normal Cal	Normal Cal

Chapter 7

Supplements

Many useful supplements are advertised today, but if you are tempted to use all of them, resist that lure. Your body will not be able to handle the load. On the other hand, there is no one perfect supplement. So in this book, we concentrate on those that have been proven effective.

The claims of some supplement distributors have not been proven. In many instances, the swimsuit models displayed in the advertising pictures have never used the product. The effects claimed were never statistically proven. One case deals with Human Growth Hormone substances that stimulate the glands. The public may be misled by the anti-aging benefits the advertiser boasts about. Usually the distributor fails to mention that these benefits were registered when the Human Growth Hormone was given by injection in extremely high dosages.

Another example of a supplement that is not effective is Pyruvate. To get results, the dosage should be up to 10 grams a day or forty 250-mg tabs, which makes it not cost effective.

The list of ineffective and useless supplements could fill a book as thick as *Harry Potter*, so let's concentrate on the useful ones.

Metabolism Boosters

It is difficult to find a supplement that will raise the rate of your basal metabolism although many product labels claim that they increase metabolism. As noted, the rate of your basal metabolism directly correlates with your age and is affected by the levels of Human Growth Hormone, sex hormones and thyroid hormones in your blood. The older you get, the lower the hormone level, and the slower your basal metabolism.

Human Growth Hormone Somatotropin

Human Growth Hormone is a hormone you can use to fight fat. It gets to the root of the problem by increasing the rate of basal metabolism and provides additional anti-aging benefits.

HGH is a large molecule, similar in size to insulin, which cannot be absorbed through membranes. So Human Growth Hormone is taken as injections. They are safe and have been used effectively for years by professional athletes. HGH is expensive, starting at $200 a month.

The natural way to increase Human Growth Hormone secretion is through exercise. Studies have shown that the more intense the exercise, the more HGH and other anabolic hormones are released. Even elderly people show increased levels of these hormones after intense exercise[78]. Please see Max Effort exercise in Part II.

Human Growth Hormone Secretagoges

Secretagoges are substances meant to stimulate internal gland functions, such as that involved in releasing Human Growth Hormone. Many commercial products sold in health food stores and on the Internet claim they can increase your Human Growth Hormone level by up to 400 percent. In truth, they cannot.

Even though some people report sleep improvement and some other effects after using commercial products, these effects are attributed to relaxing action of L-arginine on blood vessels. (L-arginine is an amino-acid, usually is a part of a secretagoge's blend)

Experiments show that some amino acids and L-dopa increase Human Growth Hormone levels in the blood if taken as injections in large doses over a short period of time. The effects are not the same if taking orally and in long term usage.

The effects of orally administered drugs are different from intravenous or intramuscular injection. To achieve an effective level in the blood, the oral dosage should be two to three times higher than the intravenous dosage. That's because it undergoes liver detoxification before it reaches the tissues. One recent publication reported that high intravenous doses of L-arginine (4 gm.) stimulated Human Growth Hormone secretion in some young athletes. This effect was not noticed in older people. This is how the secretagoge boom started. In order to achieve this concentration (4 gm. of L-arginine in the blood), a person would have to ingest 12 grams of Arginine powder [24 capsules of 500 mg each]. In addition, over time the stimulating action would tend to subside because the body adjusts to stimulation. The bottom line is: Human Growth Hormone secretagoges are not practical.

DHEA vs. 7 Keto

This hormone is produced by the adrenal glands. It is the precursor of all sex hormones. As we age, the secretion of DHEA declines leading to a decline of sex hormone production. Supplementing DHEA seemingly would be an effective way to restore the level of sex hormones, but I don't recommend the use of DHEA. It increases both testosterone and estrogen and it may lead to gynecomastia, which translates in men as breast gland enlargement and for women an increase in the risk of breast cancer.

Fortunately, there is a safe alternative – 7-Keto (available from Now Foods Inc.). It is a byproduct of DHEA conversion. It has not been converted into sex hormones, but it does effectively increase anabolism. Studies report that its use leads to significant fat loss accompanied by an increase in both energy and metabolism. There are no negative side effects reported even at high dosages. I recommend one 25-mg tablet after breakfast or one hour before exercise.

Avoid Thyroid Hormone

The thyroid hormone provides a great short-term effect but has negative long-term consequences. Because this hormone increases the rate of the metabolism, fat loss is rapid. If you take a thyroid hormone for longer than three weeks, your own Thyroid Stimulating Hormone will become suppressed and take a long time to return to normal state. This hormone should be used under a physician's supervision only.

L- Tyrosine

L- Tyrosine is a key amino acid in thyroid hormone synthesis. It is a precursor of thyroxine, a thyroid hormone, as well as the neurotransmitters adrenaline and noradrenaline.

Patients with a thyroxine deficiency experience excess weight gain, depression, cold hands and feet, difficulty concentrating and a decreased basal metabolism. L-Tyrosine supplementation might restore the thyroxine level to normal. The recommended daily dosage is 500 mg to 1,500 mg.

Kelp for Iodine

Kelp is a source of iodine. Combined with L-Tyrosine it forms a thyroid hormone. Take one capsule of kelp with one capsule of L-Tyrosine (500 mg) every other day in the morning during a three-week course. Do not exceed the recommended dosage of kelp because heart palpitations and sleep disturbance may result.

Energy-Increasing Supplements

Caffeine

Caffeine, a well-known stimulant in the athletic world, has been proven to be safe even in high doses[47,48,49]. Professional bodybuilders use it before their workout sessions to increase exercise performance and bring workout intensity to the highest possible level. This allows them to achieve the workload level at which a muscle's myofibrils become torn.

Although recreational enthusiasts are often advised to abstain from consuming caffeinated beverages, studies indicate that it stimulates exercise performance with a mild diuretic effect. There was no evidence of fluid-electrolyte imbalances or any other health hazards[47,48,49].

A daily intake of caffeine equal to five cups of coffee in one sitting (less than 500 mg. caffeine) has no side effects. With regular consumption of caffeine, a person may develop a tolerance to many of its effects.

DMAE

Dimethylaminoethanol (DMAE) is another safe and effective supplement that increases energy levels. DMAE, a natural substance produced in the brain, is involved in the synthesis of acetylcholine. It also improves mental functioning. Take one capsule in the morning together with one capsule of kelp and one of L-Tyrosine. Add Vitamin B-Complex (B-50 from Now). These vitamins are important for improved energy production.

Note: If you have elevated blood pressure do not use this combination. Use Coenzyme Q10 and NADH instead.

Coenzyme Q10

Coenzyme Q10 is essential for the production of the high-energy phosphate, adenosine triphosphate (ATP). Coenzyme Q10 is an excellent antioxidant, which means it will bond with the free radical molecules formed because of increased oxygen turnover during aerobic exercises[38]. Free radicals are molecules responsible for developing more than 80 diseases, including heart disease, cancer, arthritis and the neurodegenerative disease of aging. The effective daily dose for coenzyme Q10 is 120 to 1,000 mg. This ability to deliver both increased endurance and protection from free radicals makes it the best supplement to take when doing aerobic exercise.

NADH (Nicotinamide Adenine Dinucleotide)

NADH is the principal carrier of electrons in the oxidation of molecules that produce energy in the body's cells. It is the body's most powerful antioxidant and is 300 times more powerful than Vitamin E or C. Like Q10, it increases energy levels and provides protection from free radicals, making it another good supplement to take when doing aerobic exercise.

Creatine Monohydrate

There's *a lot* of buzz about creatine. We hear about it on the news, read about it in the press and on the Net, and see it sold in stores. But just what *is* it? And why is it the number one selling supplement among athletes?

Technically, creatine is the combination of amino acids which occur naturally in the body. It's therefore a *natural compound* that delivers energy to ATP molecules. What does this supplement do? Creatine (in the form of phosphocreatine) has a number of roles to play in energy metabolism during exercise: first it acts to buffer changes in levels of muscle ATP as the body moves between rest and exercise; secondly, during more intense exercise it helps supply ATP to the working muscles; thirdly, it helps to control pH levels in exercising muscles. The store of phosphocreatine within the muscle is relatively small, so during high-intensity exercise there is only enough to support ATP production for a few seconds.

How does creatine benefit performance? The vast majority of research points to the conclusion that supplementation with creatine may enhance performance in activities involving short bouts of high-intensity exercise -- especially those of a repetitive nature. Boosting muscle phosphocreatine by means of supplementation has been shown to improve sprint-based performance in such activities as swimming, running and cycling. Benefits have also been reported for resistance exercise. Once you know how creatine might -- and cannot -- help, you can decide whether it would be helpful to support your particular training goal.

Does supplementation lead to side effects? There are some reports of adverse effects, including fatigue, vomiting, stomach cramps and anxiety. But much of the evidence for these effects is anecdotal and, as yet, there is no proof that they are actually caused by taking creatine.

As you can see, the *more* ATP, the more energy to be released, and the longer the muscles can work without any shortages in energy supply. In a nutshell, creatine supplementation increases endurance and tolerance for all athletic activity, but particularly for high intensity exercises. In other words, individuals will typically be able to run longer, push heavier weights, feel more energetic, and achieve training goals with the aid of creatine. Remember, though: creatine is not the type of supplement that gives an instant energy boost. Its effect is accumulative, which means that it develops over time.

I recommend taking 1.5 - 3.0 grams of Creatine Monohydrate before going to sleep. Why? Because you can experience *twice* the benefits. Aside from helping you feed your muscles with energy, creatine stimulates the pituitary gland to release more Human Growth

Hormone (HGH). As a result, you'll feel more energetic and refreshed next morning. As an alternative option take it 60 minutes before exercise. The recent study shows that if creatine is taken before exercise it helps to stimulate muscle growth and accelerates recovery.

Lecithin

Lecithin is the most abundant phospholipid serving as a structural material for every cell in the body and is an essential constituent of the brain and nervous system responsible for breaking down cholesterol, transporting fats, rebuilding organs, maintaining organ, cardiovascular, and endocrine health. It fights infections, lowers blood pressure, restores sexual energy, eases PMS and menopausal tension, promotes energy and benefits nervous and mental disorders. It will also diminish post –exercise muscle and joint pains since provides needed material for cell's recovery. I recommend taking 2 tablespoons 1 hour before the exercise session or mix it with your whey protein drink and drink it right after.

Limited Roles for Diet Pills

Everyone who is trying to lose weight faces the question, "Are those pills really effective and should I use them or not?" These kinds of supplements (Hydroxycut, Xenadrine, etc) deliver appetite suppression and provide an increase in energy level. When used alone they can be considered as a temporary solution to permanent problem. I advise my patients to rely on these pills in two scenarios only:

1. In the beginning of a diet program when your behavior is changing, but insulin secretion has not yet adjusted to the smaller amounts of food you eat;

2. Occasional, short-term usage when breaking through a plateau.

When Can You Expect Results ?

Be realistic. Do not expect to see changes overnight. Be persistent and disciplined. That will assure results. The first noticeable results start to appear after a month.

Last Words

A few words before I lay down my pen.

Calorie Cycling gives you the luxury of eating forbidden foods. In return you need to make an effort to be disciplined. Is it difficult? Think about people on the Atkins diet. They are denied French fries and mom's cake — for the rest of their lives.

Be disciplined. Do not jump from one regimen to another. Do so only after restudying the instructions in this book. Give yourself time; learn from your mistakes. If you do not see results within four weeks, do not become disappointed; learn and learn to adjust.

And remember that exercise makes a huge difference. Even a short time spent exercising is better than none.

❖ ❖ ❖

Part IV

For Those Who Don't Exercise

First of all, let's make it clear. You are bringing up the rear. You are in the least advantaged group. You are the awkward squad. You may have reasons for not exercising. But are they valid reasons? Is it lack of time or is it lethargy?

Exercise provides long list of anti-aging and disease prevention benefits. If performed regularly it will revive and renew your life, bring more energy and excitement into your days. Why do some people hate gyms and exercise? Probably because they don't know about the advantages of exercise or they simply prefer to grow with the other couch potatoes.

Some people want to resist nature's summons for aging and diseases. These are people who want to take every step they can to delay age-related disability and diseases. Diet and exercise are the two easiest, cheapest and most important factors in the arsenal of weapons against aging. The heart is the muscle that moves blood through the arteries and vessels. As we age the heart's strength diminishes – the heart's output falters. The organs receive less blood and fewer nutrients, opening the gateway for degenerative conditions to take control.

What is the obvious preventive solution? Keep the heart pumping blood at an accelerated rate every day. That way it remains strong and powerful. That means exercise. It's not just a matter of increased circulation. Faster heart action means more nutrients and anti-oxidants are delivered to the organs, including the skin, which is an organ. Exercise increases the strength and activity of cells responsible for fighting cancer.

Is it possible to lose fat without exercise? Yes, it is. An important qualifier: It is almost impossible to get rid of problem-area fat — love handles, thick thighs, big butt — without a well-conceived exercise program. Exercise is an important support factor but diet is the main element in losing fat.

If you are not a physically active person, your daily calorie requirement is very close to your BMR (Basal Metabolic Rate). If you have a desk job, the number of calories you burn is about the same as when you sleep. That makes your Daily Calorie Needs almost equal to BMR. What is Daily Calorie Needs? It is the amount of calories your body needs to sustain optimum health. You will not lose fat if eat the Daily Calorie Needs of calories.

The most difficult part is not to slide backwards. That is why exercise is important .

Let's see if you can squeeze in some sort of physical activity. Can you walk home? Get off the bus two or three stops before your regular stop and walk home fast. Monitor your time and compete with yourself. Try to improve your timing every week. Can you take the stairs instead of an escalator or elevator?

Where there is a will, there is a way. What we have just described is not a big exercise program, but it is certainly better than nothing. Best of all, you might set your mind in the right direction.

Should You Count Calories?

Few people want to bother with counting calories. Let me give you some sage advice: do it , especially in the beginning. The calculation of calorie balance gives a guideline and understanding of the metabolic condition of your body. If the balance is negative – catabolism — expect a fat loss. If it is equal to your daily calorie requirements, expect no fat loss but you can count on effective protein metabolism. Start a food diary and record the number of calories consumed daily. In two to three months, you will learn the calorie values of various foods and there will no longer be a need to keep a diary.

The error in calorie calculation is almost always high, sometimes giving the user an impression that he or she has a calorie deficit when in reality they do not. Many times patients tell me, "I use online software to count calories. I eat 1,500 calories a day, and burn 2,000, but do not see a fat loss." Several factors play a role here, Let's review the numbers. The technology is evolving but we still rely a century-old formula for calculating the BMR. This formula allows up to 13 percent error in calculation. When a patient tells me he or she burns 2,000 calories a day, I adjust that to about 1,700.

Another thing to consider: Do you know that the calorie numbers for fat, protein and carbohydrates were measured by burning them to ash in a calorimeter? That destructive action takes place outside the human body. Inside the body, the calorie-burning process is quite different. It does not leave ash as an end-product of oxidation. We still need to learn how it is done in the human body.

❖ ❖ ❖

Part V

How to Start an Exercise Program

It takes time to build endurance and stamina. You may run for three months before noticing any improvement. The mistake many people make is that they expect to see stamina improvement right up front, early in the game. When they do not see it, they become disappointed and question the program's effectiveness. Or they drop the exercise program altogether.

In the beginning, during your first year, do not make intensity your primary goal. Instead, your goals should be:

1. Set a routine for regular exercising

2. Establish the number of miles run or walked each week.

3. Concentrate on the number of breaks you take during an exercise session.

For example, set a reasonable number of miles you can run or walk each day. Let's say 5K. That's three miles. With an 18-inch stride, that's 10,000 steps — precisely the number that exercise gurus regard as a daily minimum to maintain good health. No matter if you feel energetic or not, no matter how many stops you make, you should complete that 5K (three miles) every time you exercise.

Some people use another approach. On days when they lack the energy for an extended run they make shorter runs. I tell them, "No matter how, you do it, you should cross that imaginary finish line. You can make 10 brief rest stops. You can walk, run, walk, run. It is important to complete your daily, weekly and monthly miles. It is important to make exercise a routine. A 5K every day is a thousand miles a year — and an all-new you.

As a training goal, eliminate one break each month. When the number of breaks is down to one, use one training session each week to run the distance non-stop. Yes, you can run slowly — just complete the task — that 5K which appeared impossible a few months ago. Once your running routine is established, allocate one or two days a week to do interval training (sprints) only. Set your target for 6 to 10 two-minute accelerations.

If you are severely overweight, running can put major stress on your ankles and knee joints. Still, walking does not burn enough calories. The solution: during the early months, put your accent on weight lifting and do your aerobics on elliptical machine. Later, when your weight comes down, initiate running sessions into your program. At first, you will need a longer recovery period along with increased supplements to support your joints. During the first few months of training, we recommend formulas containing MSM, Chondroitin sulfate, Glucosamine, Sea cucumber, Boswellia extract and Bromelain. See the shopping list at the end of the book.

■ Time yourself. Keep a personal record and try to improve it. It's possible. To beat yourself can actually be a bigger thrill than watching a tense baseball game.

Here is an example of a 1–4 cycling regimen:

Day	Mon	Tue	Wed	Thurs	Fri	Sat	Sun
Activity	Strength training	OFF	Aerobic	Aerobic	OFF	Strength training	OFF
Diet	Normal Cal	Low Cal	Low Cal	Low Cal	Low Cal	Normal Cal	Low Cal

As you become adapted to your exercise routine, increase the number of days for aerobic exercise.

Are Breaks Okay?

Running: Breaks during your run are okay if your break time does not exceed two minutes.

Weight Lifting: Breaks between repetitions during weight lifting should not exceed 40 seconds.

Doing Interval Training Correctly

Interval training is a type of exercise designed to increase the amount of time you spend exercising at high intensities. It's a stop-and-go cycle, with stops kept short. The interval time can vary but, as studies show, the most beneficial break is two minutes. A two-minute exercise interval followed by no more than two minutes rest

109

will increase your endurance and stamina. The general rule: The shorter rest time the greater the benefit.

How to Start Strength Training

For novices I recommend starting with glycogen-depleting exercises described in Chapter 6. After gaining some muscle tone and strength, start Circuit training.

Circuit Training

- For those who want to get in shape, and do

  it fast, this is a step number one.

Circuit training, for people already at a high level of fitness, involves exercising the upper and lower portions of the body on an alternating basis — with minimum rest between changes. This is done by lifting weights using dumbbells or with resistance training machines set at moderate weight. The idea is that while the arms are recovering, the legs are working, and vice versa. The goal is to give a workout to every big muscle in the body.

Circuit training may seem difficult for beginners since it requires a high level of fitness, but the benefits are outstanding. It improves muscular strength, cardiovascular system functioning and the general fitness level. People doing circuit training really feel alive. Research shows that it increases lean body mass significantly. A five- to seven-pound gain in lean body mass can be expected with a corresponding decrease in relative fat mass.

Three sequences — or circuits — are performed. The total workout can be completed in 30 to 40 minutes. Typically, 10 to 12 weight exercises are performed for the upper-body and another dozen exercises for the lower-body; There are 15 repetitions of each exercise. Allow no more than 30 seconds rest between exercises. Circuit training with rest periods of 60 seconds can blow the whole effort. While there is fat loss, there are no improvement in conditioning.

Fast and Slow Weightlifting

I recommend the following method of lifting weights:

1. Always start with low/medium weights and perform flexion movement as fast as you can – on count 1. Extend slow on count 1,2,3. Do many reps – 20 or more.

2. Perform 10 -15 sets. You should feel burning sensation in your muscles.

3. Increase weight significantly so you will be able to do only 4 reps. Do it slowly (3-5 sets).

4. Finish with 2 sets of fast movements with light weights.

Recovery After Exercise

Muscle soreness is a normal reaction of the body to physical stress. A feeling of muscle soreness is a sign that the exercise was performed properly and effectively. It means you can expect health and fat-loss benefits from it.

The rule of thumb: Increase your physical activity – increase your nutritional support. Under physical stress, the body needs more vitamins, more minerals, more amino acids. The joints need the attention of special supplementation.

To accelerate recovery after exercise, consider taking:

• Vitamin E, Vitamin C or Alpha Lipoic acid, 300 mg

• Lecithin 1,200 mg

• Calcium 1,000 mg

How to Break the Plateau

The fat-loss process is not linear. Rather it is like a garden-path stairway with long, flat flagstone steps. Sometimes it takes a lot of effort to climb one step. Many times you will spend a long time on one level and seemingly not move any further. If that happens, review your diet. Consider these suggestions:

• Review your diet. Make adjustments. For example, use Stevia Plus instead of Splenda. Decrease the fat in your diet — it has more than twice the calorie level of protein or carbohydrates. Finally, increase your use of whey protein or egg whites.

• Review your exercises. Change them. Change the times when you exercise. Split your exercises into two sessions. On weekends, adopt morning and evening sessions. Incorporate one interval (stop-and-go sprint) training session each week. Weight lifting: change the number of repetitions. Change the rest period. Start circuit training with minimum rest between exercises. Increase the intensity of your workouts. Do anything you can think of to fool your body.

The Calorie Cycling Diet was designed to prevent adaptation: the regimens are not pre-set but rather dynamic and can be changed as you go. Change them periodically and keep alternating your exercises.

To find organizations that can provide a support for novices in exercising, please refer to the Resources Section at the end of the book.

Part VI

For Those Who Exercise

Countless laboratory-based studies have demonstrated the many health and fitness benefits associated with endurance exercising. To increase your total fitness, incorporate high intensity interval training into your workouts.

To increase your total level of fitness and enjoy the benefits of this program, you need to increase your muscle mass. To increase your muscle mass, temporarily switch to Macro-cycling that was described in Chapter 6. Start with Regimen 2–3 or 3–3. For serious fitness enthusiasts, working up to a rigorous 14–14 regimen will deliver the better results.

During the normal-cal days, do weight lifting only. No aerobic exercises!

During the following protein-packed (calorie-restricted) days, do circuit training and those aerobic running and swimming exercises, which aim at conditioning the heart and lungs.

Here is a summary of medical studies showing the benefits of regular exercise.

Table 1-x

Results of Studies Investigating the Relationship Between Physical Activity or Physical Fitness and Incidences of Selected Chronic Diseases.

Disease or Condition	Strength of Evidence
All-cause mortality	⇓ ⇓ ⇓
Coronary artery disease	⇓ ⇓ ⇓
Hypertension	⇓ ⇓
Blood lipid profile change	⇓ ⇓ ⇓
Obesity	⇓ ⇓ ⇓
Stroke	⇓
Colon cancer	⇓ ⇓ ⇓
Rectal cancer	No difference
Stomach cancer	No difference
Breast cancer	⇓ ⇓
Prostate cancer	⇓
Lung cancer	⇓
Pancreas cancer	No difference
Type 2 diabetes	⇓ ⇓
Osteoarthritis	No difference
Osteoporosis	⇓ ⇓

Adapted from ACSM's Guidelines for Exercise Testing and Prescription, Sixth Edition, © 2000, Lippincott, Williams & Wilkins ISBN 0-683-30355-4

Risks Associated with Vigorous Exercise.

You are responsible for your own life. Take care of yourself but do it carefully. Increased demands for oxygen during exercise may precipitate heart and blood vessel (cardiovascular) complications in a person with heart disease. Cardiovascular problems have been reported in sedentary people who engaged in sporadic high-intensity exercise — the couch potato who becomes a roaring Tarzan on weekends. That kind of person is not physically conditioned.

I recommend that you begin slowly. Before you start, consult your physician or cardiologist and get a medical clearance. Later do a follow-up with your favorite medic. For the first year — or even two — you need to pre-condition your body by walking and circuit training. Only then can you take up high-intensity training. The risk of both cardiovascular and orthopedic injuries increases at higher intensities of physical exertion. To prevent these injuries, precede every exercise session with properly performed warm-up and stretching sessions. And take supplements that help you during exercise.

When You Stop Exercising

Numerous studies were conducted to investigate the consequences of a reduced exercise program or a complete cessation of cardio-respiratory fitness training. A significant reduction of cardiovascular fitness occurs within two weeks of stopping. Most of the reduction occurs when the intensity of training is reduced. In contrast,

decreasing the frequency or duration of daily training had little
influence — provided that the intensity was maintained. In other
words, intensity is again the key word here.

Recovery After Exercise

An increase in physical activity requires an increase in nutritional
support. Think about it for five seconds and you have to agree that
the body under physical stress needs more vitamins, minerals, amino
acids and supplements. If you are older than 40, your joints also need
special attention. To accelerate your recovery after exercise, take the
following:

Vitamin C

Vitamin E

Lecithin

Calcium

Creatine Monohydrate

Weight Lifting for Women

Many women actively shun weight lifting, fearing — needlessly —
that it will turn them into bulges of flexing muscles. That's not a
valid excuse to avoid exercise. Muscle-building requires that high
levels of anabolic hormones (testosterone) be circulating in the blood.
Since women have lower levels of testosterone, successful muscle-
building would require Herculean efforts on her part. Only one in a
thousand would undertake such a challenge.

After weight-lifting exercises, you may notice an increase in muscle size. That is attributable to three things: better blood flow, water retention and the plumping effect of muscle glycogen. These changes are not permanent. A few days after you stop weight lifting, the plumping will disappear.

The Calorie Cycling Diet is a kissing' cousin to the diet and exercise template used by professional bodybuilders and Olympic athletes. For readers of this book, the diet was adjusted for use by ordinary people — including those who do not exercise. As a result, CCD is the most powerful diet regimen known to medicine. It is an almighty tool, leaving the choice to you on how to best utilize the power of this diet for your own benefit. I made this diet flexible and adjustable for use by everyone. By switching between levels, increasing cal-restricting days and changing tactics, you can regulate the speed and extent of fat loss and muscle retention. You can adjust the regimen to the needs of your lifestyle. If you skip your morning exercise, simply make the day a low-cal one. Among the greatest benefits for some is the fact that it is possible for people who don't exercise to use the CCD and improve their bodies. You can start, stop and start over again at any time. Good luck, good health and may you live to enjoy happiness in your golden years.

Special Exercises from Dr. Malkov

I am going to show exercises that I developed as a result of many years of practicing the Cal Cycling Diet. There were days when I was unable to go to the gym and exercise there. I noticed that if muscles are "sleepy" (not active) they are not consuming many calories and have little impact on total metabolism. The Daily Calorie Needs become less than I wanted and it was easy to exceed that number of calories. So I needed to find a way of activating muscles without using any equipment. Likely I came to a solution! It all started with hemorrhoid. I developed this condition 2 years ago probably as a result of lifting a heavy weight. I started to do a special exercise to prevent it appearance- to exercise the anus muscles. These muscles close the openings of rectum. To train them you need to perform the same muscle movements as you do when finishing defecation – tighten and relax them. 6 repetitions. 10 sets. Every day. The good news is you can do it everywhere. At home. At work. In the bus. In the car. In one month of doing this exercise the muscles became stronger and hemorrhoid disappeared forever. This exercise is also good for a prostate. It increases the blood circulation in pelvic area.

I realized that any muscles can be fired up like that. So I came up to exercises that activate all body. It can be used together with yoga or on its own. It can be done in office!

Do it every time when you have a free moment:

1. Put your wrists together
2. Constrict (tighten) arms, shoulder and chest muscles and relax them. You can do it on count 1, 2 or hold it for a few seconds before relaxing.
3. Do it 10 times. Rest a few seconds. Repeat 5 times (5 sets).
4. Unlock your wrists.
5. Tighten muscles of the back and shoulder.
6. Do it 10 times. Rest a few seconds. Repeat 5 times.
7. Move to the abdominal area.
8. Tighten abdominal muscles and relax them. You will need to hold your breath while doing it.
9. Do it 10 times. Rest a few seconds. Repeat 5 times (5 sets).
10. Move to leg muscles.

11.   Bring the legs to the bottom of the table so they will not move when you tighten the muscles.
12.   Tighten the muscles and relax them.
13.   Do it 10 times. Rest a few seconds. Repeat 5 times.
Your aim is to work out as many muscles as possible, especially the big muscles. Also, repeat exercises a few times a day to keep muscles metabolically active all day long.

✠ ✠ ✠

Questions and Answers

What is Vmax?

Vmax – Maximum speed.

Do normal-cal days cause difficulties in controlling blood sugar?

No. On the first low-cal day, your insulin level quickly returns to a low value.

How do you monitor progress?

Weigh yourself every morning. One or two pounds of weight gain may be attributed to food or water retention. Three pounds of gain should alert you to take action.

What do I do, if I skip exercise?

Make the day Level B: cal-restricted.

Your CCD Shopping List

Here is a list that you may consult when you go shopping for vitamins, minerals and food supplements for the CCD diet. The names are product brands that we recommend. They are available at most health food stores.

Daily Vitamin & Mineral Supplement

• Calcium. 1,000 to 1,750 mg. 1,200 is the RDA for seniors.

• Omega-3, Omega-6, Omega-9 detoxified fish oils from Health from the Sun or Now Foods. On low-cal days, take 5-10 grams a day.

• Coenzyme Q-10, 120 to 1,000 mg. When doing aerobic exercises, Q-10 is the best supplement to take.

• NADH is 300 times more powerful than Vitamin C or E in fighting radicals. A good supplement to take when doing aerobic exercise.

Anytime as a Snack

• Whey Protein Isolate, from Now Foods

• Branched Chain Amino Acids, from Now Foods, 6 -10 capsules as a snack. Carry it with you for snacks on the go.

To Prevent Food Cravings

• Alpha Lipoic Acid, 300 mg, from Natrol

• Gymnemna Sylvestre capsules, from Now Foods

• Garcinia Cambogia capsules, from Now Foods

• L- Carnitine Liquid, to prevent cravings for sweets, from Now Foods

Energy for Muscles

• Creatine Monohydrate 1000 mg from Now Foods.

For Joint Recovery After Exercise:

• Vitamin E, Vitamin C or Alpha Lipoic acid, 300 mg

• Lecithin softgels, from CVS, 1,200 mg

• Calcium, 1,000 mg

To Increase Metabolism

7-Keto, from Now Foods Inc. One 25-mg tablet after breakfast or one hour before exercise.

Thyroid Hormone for Energy

• Kelp Caps, from Now Foods.

• L-Tyrosine. Take one capsule of kelp with one 500 mg capsule of L-Tyrosine every other day in the morning during a three-week course. Do not exceed the recommended dosage of kelp.

• DMEA, 250, mg, from Now Foods

• Vitamin B-50, from Now Foods

High Blood Pressure?

Note: If you have elevated blood pressure, do not use DMEA and Vitamin B-50. Use Coenzyme Q10 and NADH instead.

To Relieve Arthritis Pain

• Joint Support, from Now Foods.

Overweight or Obese?

Joint support formulas are recommended during the first few months of exercise. For overweight dieters, they include:

• Glucosamine

• Chondroitin sulfate

• MSM

• Sea cucumber

• Boswellia extract

• Bromelain

About the Author

Roman Malkov, M.D., is admirably qualified to write this book on weight loss and optimum health — based on the proven principles of Sports Medicine. Dr. Malkov was graduated from Moscow Medical University in 1989 as a gastroenterologist. For several years, he served as Attending Physician at Central Hospital in Moscow and as a Nutritional Consultant for the Russian National Athletic Team. In 1997, he passed the U.S. Medical License examination. He is an active member of the American Collage of Sports Medicine. His private practice is established in New York City where he is a consultant to professional athletes and fitness enthusiasts.

— finis —

www.ingramcontent.com/pod-product-compliance
Lightning Source LLC
Chambersburg PA
CBHW031520270326
41930CB00006B/458